ABC of
Arterial and Venous Disease

Second edition

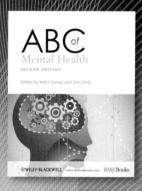
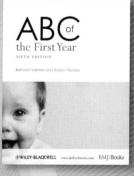
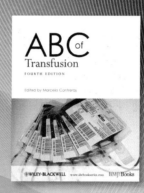
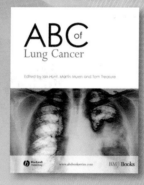
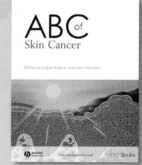
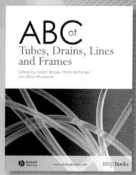

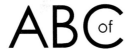

Arterial and Venous Disease

Second edition

Richard Donnelly

Professor of Vascular Medicine
School of Graduate-Entry Medicine and Health
University of Nottingham
Derby City General Hospital
Derby
UK

Nick JM London

Professor of Surgery
Leicester University
Leicester
UK

WILEY-BLACKWELL
A John Wiley & Sons, Ltd., Publication

BMJ|Books

This edition first published 2009, © 2009 by Blackwell Publishing Ltd

BMJ Books is an imprint of BMJ Publishing Group Limited, used under licence by Blackwell Publishing which was acquired by John Wiley & Sons in February 2007. Blackwell's publishing programme has been merged with Wiley's global Scientific, Technical and Medical business to form Wiley-Blackwell.

Registered office: John Wiley & Sons Ltd, The Atrium, Southern Gate, Chichester, West Sussex PO19 8SQ, UK

Editorial offices: 9600 Garsington Road, Oxford OX4 2DQ, UK
The Atrium, Southern Gate, Chichester, West Sussex PO19 8SQ, UK
111 River Street, Hoboken, NJ 07030-5774, USA

For details of our global editorial offices, for customer services and for information about how to apply for permission to reuse the copyright material in this book please see our website at www.wiley.com/wiley-blackwell

The right of the author to be identified as the author of this work has been asserted in accordance with the Copyright, Designs and Patents Act 1988.

Library of Congress Cataloging-in-Publication Data
ABC of arterial and venous disease / [edited by] Richard Donnelly, Nick JM London. – 2nd ed.
       p. ; cm. – (ABC series)
    Includes bibliographical references and index.
    ISBN 978-1-4051-7889-1
    1. Blood-vessels–Diseases.   I. Donnelly, Richard, 1960–   II. London, Nick J. M.
III. Series: ABC series (Malden, Mass.)
    [DNLM: 1. Vascular Diseases–diagnosis.   2. Vascular Diseases–therapy.
WG 500 A133 2009]
    RC691.A23 2009
    616.1′3–dc22

                                                          2008052025

ISBN: 978-1-4051-7889-1

A catalogue record for this book is available from the British Library.

Set in 9.25/12 pt Minion by SNP Best-set Typesetter Ltd., Hong Kong
Printed & bound in Singapore by Ho Printing Singapore Pte Ltd

2   2010

Contents

Preface

The clinical manifestations of arterial and venous disease are often the result of various pathophysiological mechanisms, including atherosclerosis, thrombosis, inflammation, embolism and aneurysm formation. Recent developments in non-invasive imaging particularly duplex scanning, high resolution CT and magnetic resonance imaging have revolutionised the identification of structural and functional abnormalities in arteries and veins.

There have been significant changes in our knowledge of arterial and venous diseases since the last edition of this book in 2000. This revised and updated edition is designed to provide a contemporary and practical description of the techniques used to diagnose, investigate and manage arterial and venous diseases. The authorship reflects an integrated approach to clinical management involving surgeons, physicians, radiologists and vascular laboratory technicians working closely to achieve optimum outcomes. For example, the approach to carotid disease and renal artery stenosis demonstrates the importance of multidisciplinary input to clinical decision making.

This book is targeted primary at the non-specialist and wherever possible, we have tried to ensure that clinical practice recommendations in this book are evidence based. However, clinical trials in patients with arterial and venous disease are relatively limited and there remain gaps in our knowledge. Nevertheless, we hope that this book provides an up-to-date text covering best practice in a rapidly changing and diverse group of common clinical disorders.

Richard Donnelly
University of Nottingham
Nick JM London
University of Leicester

Contributors

William D Adair
Consultant Radiologist, Department of Vascular and Endovascular Surgery, Leicester Royal Infirmary, Leicester, UK

Ali Arshad
Speciality Registrar in Vascular Surgery, Leicester Royal Infirmary, Leicester, UK

Amman Bolia
Consultant Vascular Radiologist, Department of Vascular and Endovascular Surgery, Leicester Royal Infirmary, Leicester, UK

Matthew J Bown
Lecturer in Surgery, University of Leicester, Leicester, UK

Adrian J Brady
Department of Medical Cardiology, Glasgow Royal Infirmary, Glasgow, UK

Julie Brittenden
Reader in Surgery, Aberdeen University, Aberdeen, UK

Martin JS Dennis
Consultant Vascular Surgeon, Department of Vascular and Endovascular Surgery, Leicester Royal Infirmary, Leicester, UK

Mario De Nunzio
Consultant Radiologist, Derby Hospitals NHS Foundation Trust, Derby, UK

Richard Donnelly
Professor of Vascular Medicine, School of Graduate-Entry Medicine and Health, University of Nottingham, Derby City General Hospital, Derby, UK

Guy Fishwick
Consultant Radiologist, Leicester Royal Infirmary, Leicester, UK

Gary A Ford
Professor of Pharmacology of Old Age, Institute for Ageing & Health, Newcastle-Upon-Tyne NHS Foundation Trust and Newcastle University, Clinical Research Centre, Royal Victoria Infirmary, Newcastle-Upon-Tyne, UK

Manj S Gohel
Department of Vascular Surgery, Cheltenham General Hospital, Cheltenham, UK

Peter Gorman
Consultant Physician, Derby Hospitals NHS Foundation Trust, Derby, UK

Louise S Haine
Derbyshire Royal Infirmary, Derby, UK

Alan G Jardine
BHF Glasgow Cardiovascular Research Centre, University of Glasgow, Glasgow, UK

Vaughan Keeley
Consultant in Palliative Medicine, Derby Hospitals NHS Foundation Trust, Derby, UK

P Kesteven
Northern Vascular Unit, Freeman Hospital, Newcastle-upon-Tyne, UK

Nick JM London
Professor of Surgery, Leicester University, Leicester, UK

Patrick B Mark
Department of Renal Medicine, Western Infirmary, Glasgow, UK

Mark McCarthy
Consultant Vascular and Endovascular Surgeon, Leicester Royal Infirmary, Leicester, UK

DP Mikhailidis
Northern Vascular Unit, Freeman Hospital, Newcastle-upon-Tyne, UK

Matthew D Morgan
Division of Immunity and Infection, The Medical School, University of Birmingham, Birmingham, UK

Akhtar Nasim
Consultant Vascular Surgeon/Honorary Senior Lecturer, Leicester Royal Infirmary, Leicester, UK

A Ross Naylor
Professor of Vascular Surgery, Department of Surgery, Leicester Royal Infirmary, Leicester, UK

John Pasi
Professor of Haemostasis and Thrombosis, Centre for Haematology, Institute of Cell and Molecular Science, Barts and The London School of Medicine and Dentistry, London, UK

Keith R Poskitt

Consultant Surgeon, Cheltenham General Hospital, Cheltenham, UK

Christopher I Price

Clinical Senior Lecturer in Medicine, Northumbria Healthcare NHS Trust, Wansbeck General Hospital, Ashington, UK

Giles H Roditi

Department of Radiology, Glasgow Royal Infirmary, Glasgow, UK

Timothy E Rowlands

Consultant Vascular Surgeon, Derbyshire Royal Infirmary, Derby, UK

Caroline OS Savage

Division of Immunity and Infection, The Medical School, University of Birmingham, Birmingham, UK

Robert D Sayers

Professor of Vascular Surgery, University of Leicester, Leicester, UK

Stuart W Smith

Division of Immunity and Infection, The Medical School, University of Birmingham, Birmingham, UK

G Stansby

Professor of Vascular Surgery, Northern Vascular Unit, Freeman Hospital, Newcastle-upon-Tyne, UK

Garry Tan

School of Graduate-Entry Medicine and Health, Derby City General Hospital, Derby, UK

CHAPTER 1

Methods of Arterial and Venous Assessment

Peter Gorman, Mario De Nunzio, Richard Donnelly

OVERVIEW

- This chapter describes the main investigative techniques used in arterial and venous disease.
- The ankle–brachial pressure index (ABPI), calculated from the ratio of ankle systolic blood pressure (SBP) to brachial SBP, is a sensitive marker of arterial insufficiency in the lower limb, and correlates with survival.
- Blood velocity increases through an area of narrowing. Typically, a 2-fold increase in peak systolic velocity compared with the velocity in a proximal adjacent segment of the same artery usually signifies a stenosis of 50% or more.
- In detecting femoral and popliteal artery disease, duplex ultrasonography has a sensitivity of 80% and a specificity of 90–100%.
- The introduction of multidetector computed tomography (MDCT) has had a dramatic effect on vascular imaging. CT pulmonary angiography (CTPA) for suspected pulmonary embolism is a good example, but CT angiography and magnetic resonance angiography are widely used to investigate large artery pathology.
- Colour duplex scanning is both sensitive and specific (90–100% in most series) for detecting proximal deep-vein thrombosis (DVT).

Diagnostic and therapeutic decisions in patients with vascular disease are guided primarily by the history and physical examination. However, the accuracy and accessibility of non-invasive investigations have greatly increased due to technological advances in computed tomography (CT) and magnetic resonance (MR) scanning. CT angiography (CTA) and MR angiography (MRA) continue to evolve rapidly, and are best described as 'minimally invasive' techniques when used with intravenous (i.v) contrast. This chapter describes the main investigative techniques used in arterial and venous disease.

ABC of Arterial & Venous Disease, 2nd edn. Edited by R. Donnelly and N. London.
© 2009 Blackwell Publishing Ltd. 9781405178891.

Principles of vascular ultrasound

In its simplest form, ultrasound is transmitted as a continuous beam from a probe that contains two piezoelectric crystals. The transmitting crystal produces ultrasound at a fixed frequency (set by the operator according to the depth of the vessel being examined) whilst the receiving crystal vibrates in response to reflected waves and produces an output voltage. Conventional B-mode (brightness mode) ultrasonography records the ultrasound waves reflected from tissue interfaces and a two-dimensional picture is built up according to the reflective properties of the tissues.

Ultrasound signals reflected off stationary surfaces have the same frequency with which they were transmitted, but the principle underlying Doppler ultrasonography is that signals reflected from moving objects, e.g. red blood cells, undergo a frequency shift in proportion to the velocity of the target. The output from a continuous-wave Doppler ultrasound is most frequently presented as an audible signal (e.g. a hand-held pencil Doppler, Figure 1.1), so that a sound is heard whenever there is movement of blood in the vessel being examined. With continuous-wave ultrasonography there is little scope for restricting the area of tissue that is being examined because any sound waves that are intercepted by the receiving crystal will produce an output signal. The solution is to use pulsed ultrasound. This enables the investigator to focus on a specific tissue plane by transmitting a pulse of ultrasound and closing the receiver except when signals from a predetermined depth are returning. For example, the centre of an artery and the areas close to the vessel wall can be examined in turn.

Examination of an arterial stenosis shows an increase in blood velocity through the area of narrowing. The site(s) of any stenotic lesions can be identified by serial placement of the Doppler probe along the extremities. Criteria to define a stenosis vary between laboratories, but a 2-fold increase in peak systolic velocity compared with the velocity in a proximal adjacent segment of the artery usually signifies a stenosis of ≥50% (Table 1.1).

The normal ('triphasic') Doppler velocity waveform is made up of three components which correspond to different phases of arterial flow (Figure 1.2a):
- Rapid antegrade flow reaching a peak during systole
- Transient reversal of flow during early diastole
- Slow antegrade flow during late diastole.

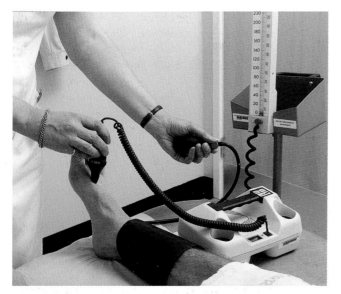

Figure 1.1 A hand-held pencil Doppler being used to measure the ankle–brachial pressure index

Table 1.1 Relationship between increased blood velocity and degree of stenosis

Diameter of stenosis (%)	Peak systolic velocity* (m/s)	Peak diastolic velocity* (m/s)	Internal common carotid artery velocity ratio†
0–39	<1.1	<0.45	<1.8
4–59	1.1–1.49	<0.45	<1.8
60–79	1.5–2.49	0.45–1.4	1.8–3.7
80–99	2.5–6.1	>1.4	>3.7
>99 (critical)	Extremely low	NA	NA

*Measured in lower part of internal carotid artery.
†Ratio of peak systolic velocity in internal carotid artery stenosis relative to proximal measurement in common carotid artery.

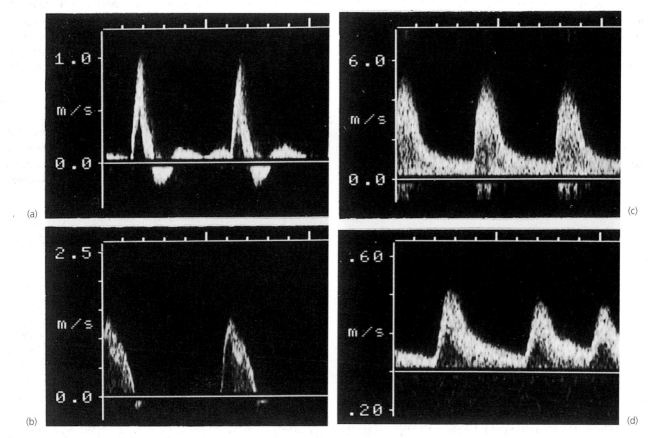

Figure 1.2 Left: Doppler velocity waveforms: (a) a triphasic waveform in a normal artery; (b) a biphasic waveform, with increased velocity, through a mild stenosis; (c) a monophasic waveform, with a marked increase in velocity, through a tight stenosis; and (d) a dampened monophasic waveform, with reduced velocity, recorded distal to a tight stenosis. Right: the results of a routine lower limb Doppler examination are typically recorded on an anatomical chart, as shown, where three stenoses are identified with velocity increases of 7×, 3× and 4× that in adjacent unaffected segments of the respective arteries

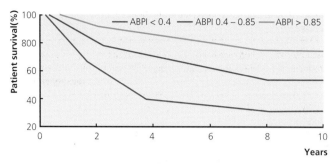

Figure 1.3 Patient survival according to measurements of ABPI. This reflects the association between peripheral arterial disease and occlusive disease in other vascular territories, especially the brain and heart (adapted from McKenna *et al.*, 1991)

Doppler examination of an artery distal to a stenosis shows characteristic changes in the velocity profile (Figure 1.2d):
- The rate of rise is delayed and the amplitude decreased
- The transient flow reversal in early diastole is lost
- In severe disease, the Doppler waveform flattens; in critical limb ischaemia, it may be undetectable.

Investigations of arterial disease

Ankle–brachial pressure index
Under normal conditions, systolic blood pressure (SBP) in the legs is equal to or slightly greater than the SBP in the upper limbs. In the presence of an arterial stenosis, a reduction in pressure occurs distal to the lesion. The ankle–brachial pressure index (ABPI), calculated from the ratio of ankle SBP to brachial SBP, is a sensitive marker of arterial insufficiency in the lower limb, and correlates with survival (Figure 1.3). The highest pressure measured in any ankle artery is used as the numerator in the calculation of the ABPI (Figure 1.3). An ABPI of ≥1.0 is normal and a value <0.9 is abnormal. Patients with claudication tend to have ABPIs in the range 0.5–0.9, whilst those with critical ischaemia usually have an index of <0.5. In patients with diabetes (in whom distal vessels are often calcified and incompressible), SBP measured in the lower limbs may be less reliable, which can result in falsely high ankle pressures and a falsely elevated ABPI.

Exercise testing will assess the functional limitations of arterial stenoses and differentiate occlusive arterial disease from other causes of exercise-induced lower limb symptoms, e.g neurogenic claudication secondary to spinal stenosis. A limited inflow of blood in a limb with occlusive arterial disease results in a fall in ankle SBP during exercise-induced peripheral vasodilatation. Patients can be exercised for 5 min, ideally on a treadmill, but walking in the surgery or marking time on the spot are perfectly adequate. ABPI is measured before and after exercise. A pressure drop of ≥20% indicates significant arterial disease (Figure 1.4). If there is no drop in ankle SBP after a 5 min brisk walk, the patient does not have occlusive arterial disease proximal to the ankle in that limb.

Duplex scanning
By combining the pulsed Doppler system with real-time B-mode ultrasound imaging of vessels, it is possible to examine (or 'sample') Doppler flow patterns in a precisely defined area within the vessel lumen. This combination of real-time B-mode sound imaging with pulsed Doppler ultrasound is called duplex scanning. The addition of colour frequency mapping makes the identification of arterial stenoses even easier and reduces scanning time (Figure 1.5).

In detecting femoral and popliteal disease, duplex ultrasonography has a sensitivity of 80% and a specificity of 90–100% but ultrasound is less reliable for assessing the severity of stenoses in the tibial and peroneal arteries (Table 1.2). Duplex scanning is especially useful for assessing the carotid arteries and for routine surveillance of infrainguinal bypass grafts where sites of stenosis can be identified before complete graft occlusion occurs and before there is a significant fall in ABPI. The normal velocity within a graft conduit ranges between 50 and 120 cm/s. As with native arteries, a 2-fold increase in peak systolic velocity indicates a stenosis of ≥50%. A peak velocity <45 cm/s occurs in grafts at high risk of failure.

Transcranial Doppler
Lower frequency Doppler probes (1–2 MHz) can be used to obtain a dynamic measurement of relative blood flow and detection of microemboli in arteries comprising the Circle of Willis and its principal branches (Box 1.1). It enables blood flow assessment and

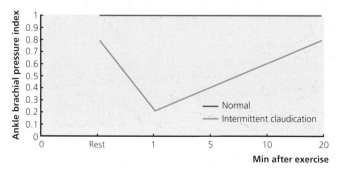

Figure 1.4 The fall in ABPI with exercise in a patient with intermittent claudication

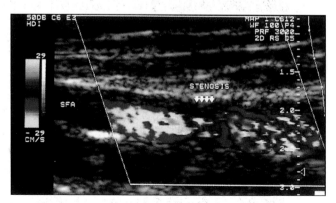

Figure 1.5 Colour duplex scanning of blood flow through a stenosis of the superficial femoral artery (SFA). The colour assignment (red or blue) depends on the direction of blood flow, and colour saturation reflects velocity of blood flow. Less saturation (red, blue) indicates regions of higher blood flow, and deeper colours indicate slower flow; the absence of flow is coded as black

Table 1.2 Uses of colour duplex scanning

Arterial	Venous

Identify obstructive atherosclerotic disease:
  Carotid
  Renal
Surveillance of infrainguinal bypass grafts
Surveillance of lower limb arteries after angioplasty
	Diagnosis of deep-vein thrombosis above the knee
	Assessing competence of valves in deep veins
	Superficial venous reflux:
	  Assessing patient with recurrent varicose veins
	  Identify and locate reflux at saphenopopliteal junction
	  Pre-operative mapping of saphenous vein

Box 1.1 Clinical uses of transcranial Doppler scanning in adults

Ischaemic cerebrovascular disease:
- stenosis and occlusion in intracranial and extracranial carotid and vertebrobasilar arteries
- collateral flow
- detection of microemboli, including from patent foramen ovale
- monitoring flow after cerebral thrombolysis

Peri-operative monitoring in carotid endarterectomy and angioplasty

Detection of vasospasm after subarachnoid haemorrhage

Evaluation of vasomotor reactivity

monitoring in a number of applications, particularly carotid endarterectomy.

Computed tomography angiography

Helical or spiral CTA is a technique that allows rapid and continuous acquisition of a helical 'ribbon' of data during the first pass of a bolus of i.v. contrast through the arterial tree. The data can be reconstructed at any slice level, reformatted into different planes and processed into high-quality two- or three-dimensional images of vessels. The introduction of multidetector CT (MDCT) has had a dramatic effect on CT imaging, and in particular imaging of the cardiovascular system. There are two main differences between conventional spiral CT and MDCT. First, MDCT has a much higher speed of data acquisition (0.37 s rotation speed versus 1 s rotation speed for conventional CT), and secondly MDCT acquires volume data instead of individual slice data. Thus, MDCT (without increas-

ing the radiation dose) has led to faster scanning, improved contrast resolution and better spatial resolution. The effect of movement artefacts is also minimized.

The time taken to complete the procedure is determined by practicalities such as moving the patient and gaining venous access, but the scan acquisition time for the entire arterial system (aortic arch to pedal vessels) is <45 s for CTA compared with ~4–5 min for MRA (Table 1.3).

Magnetic resonance angiography

MR scanning allows the use of a pulse sequence which images moving blood, thus showing arteries or veins without the use of an injected contrast agent or exposure to ionizing radiation. Non-contrast MRA therefore has substantial safety advantages but is characterized by flow dependence. Contrast-enhanced MRA using

Table 1.3 Advantages and limitations of CT and MR angiography

CTA	MRA (non-contrast/+ i.v gadolinium)
Rapid data acquisition; less prone to movement artefact	Slower; more prone to movement artefact
High-resolution images	Lower resolution but dependent on technique and location
Anatomical image of contrast in vessel	Flow dependent (non-contrast MRA)
Loss of accuracy with circumferential calcification	May indicate flow direction
	May overestimate degree and length of stenosis, due to signal dropout in areas of turbulence
Ease of access, especially in emergency context	Scanners less available
Acutely ill patients can be supported during scan	Contraindicated by need for intensive patient support
	Contraindications include implants such as pacemakers, defibrillators, cochlear implants and spinal cord stimulators
	Small scanner tunnel not tolerated by some patients due to claustrophobia or body habitus
Less expensive	More expensive
Radiation exposure	No radiation
Iodinated contrast—risk of contrast nephropathy and allergy	Non-contrast MRA is non-invasive
	Effective hydration helps prevent nephropathy, but the benefit of prophylaxis with iso-osmolar contrast agents remains controversial In contrast-enhanced MRA, gadolinium contrast has been associated with nephrogenic systemic fibrosis

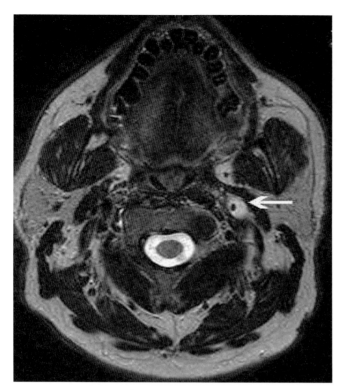

Figure 1.6 T2-weighted axial MR scan of the neck showing a left internal carotid artery dissection, with blood in the vessel wall producing a high signal (arrow)

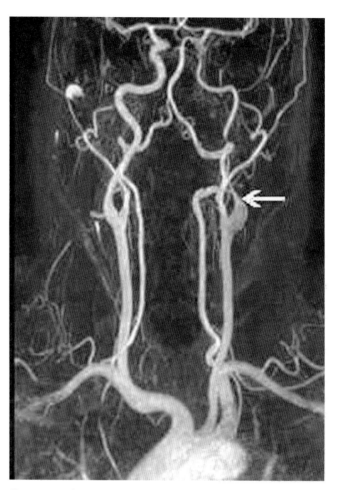

Figure 1.7 In the same patient as in Fig. 1.6, this MRA reconstruction shows a stenosis just above the origin of the left internal carotid artery (arrow)

an i.v. bolus of gadolinium contrast can cover a larger area, allows more rapid data acquisition and higher resolution, and gives a more direct image of the vascular lumen. Therefore, contrast-enhanced MRA is more commonly used, but recent advances in MR technology, partially driven by complications associated with the gadolinium-based contrast, have led to major improvements in scan quality of non-contrast MRA vascular imaging, which is likely to result in greater use in the future.

A variety of imaging sequences are used depending upon the vessels being studied and the field strength of the machine. Information is obtained both from the axial images and from vessel reconstructions (Figures 1.6 and 1.7).

Applications of CTA and MRA

CTA and MRA are both widely used to investigate large artery pathology (Figures 1.8 and 1.9). Each technique has different advantages and disadvantages (Table 1.3). CTA has the major advantage of speed, but local preferences and availability often determine which technique is used. CT pulmonary angiography (CTPA) for suspected pulmonary embolism (PE) is probably the most commonly used computerized angiographic investigation (Figure 1.10). Whereas single-detector CT shows a sensitivity of 73% and a specificity of 87% in the diagnosis of PE (based on pooled data), corresponding figures for MDCT (mostly four-slice images) are 83 and 96%. The positive predictive values for MDCT are 97% for PE in a main pulmonary artery or lobar artery, 68% for a segmental vessel and 25% for a subsegmental branch.

In abdominal aortic aneurysm (AAA) and aortic dissection imaging, CTA is the preferred investigation because it images the vessel wall and can provide information about mural thrombus, inflammatory changes and rupture. Software reconstructs hundreds of images and displays them in two- or three-dimensional planes (Figures 1.11 and 1.12). This becomes a powerful tool for pre-operative planning and post-operative follow-up, especially in regard to use of endovascular stent grafts for AAA repair. CTA is more sensitive and specific than conventional angiography in detecting the presence of endoleaks.

MDCT angiography and MRA have equally high sensitivity and specificity for the detection of renal artery stenosis, but CTA is often preferred in order to avoid gadolinium administration, especially in patients with renal impairment (Figure 1.9). MDCT can also be used post-stenting to assess for recurrent renal artery stenosis.

Some centres prefer to use MRA to image lower limb vascular disease due to the adverse effect of heavy circumferential calcification which, when using CTA, can limit accuracy and make interpretation more difficult. However, CTA has several advantages in peripheral arterial disease, e.g. visualization of extraluminal pathology, including aneurysms, better assessment of eccentric lesions and visualization of more arterial segments, particularly in occlusive disease where there is little or no flow.

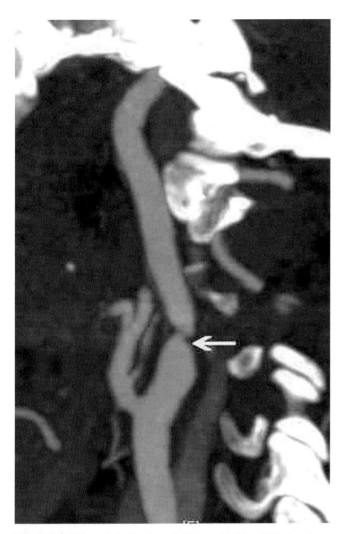

Figure 1.8 CT angiogram showing a tight stenosis of the right internal carotid artery (arrow)

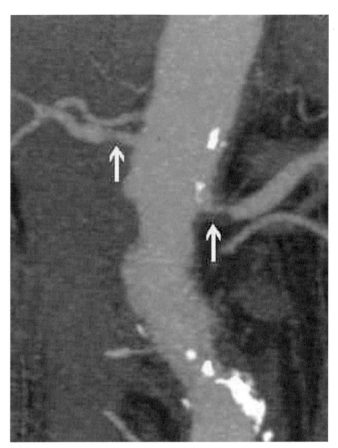

Figure 1.9 CT angiogram showing bilateral renal artery stenoses (arrows)

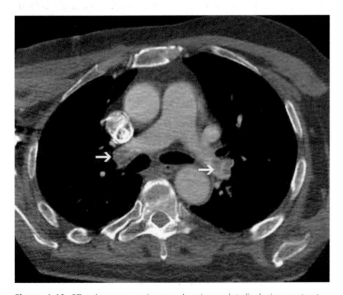

Figure 1.10 CT pulmonary angiogram showing a clot displacing contrast in both main pulmonary arteries (arrows)

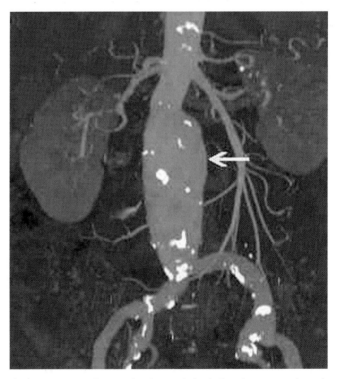

Figure 1.11 CT angiogram showing an abdominal aortic aneurysm (arrow)

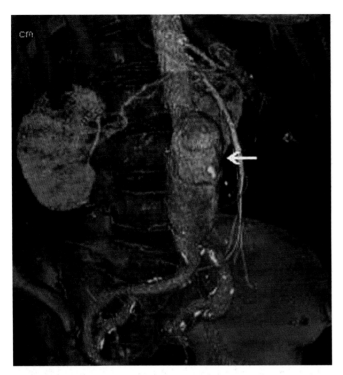

Figure 1.12 Volume-rendered reconstruction of the CT angiogram in the same patient as Fig. 1.11 (abdominal aortic aneurysm) (arrow)

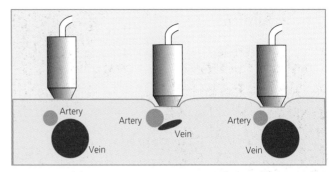

Figure 1.13 Ultrasound detection of a DVT. The probe is held lightly on the skin and advanced along the course of the vein (left). Pressure is applied every few centimetres by compressing the transducer head against the skin. The vein collapses during compression if no thrombus is present (middle) but not if a DVT is present (right)

In acute cerebral ischaemia, in addition to artery level information from angiography, data on parenchymal perfusion can be provided by MR diffusion–perfusion mismatch or CT blood volume–perfusion mismatch. These methods are gaining importance for predicting core infarct size and risk of progressive ischaemia, and for informing decisions about thrombolysis.

Investigations in venous disease

Venous thrombosis

Colour Duplex scanning is both sensitive and specific (90–100% in most series) for detecting proximal deep-vein thrombosis (DVT). Deep veins and arteries lie together in the leg, and the normal vein appears as an echo-free channel and is usually larger than the accompanying artery. Venous ultrasound has proved to be a very accurate method of identifying DVTs from the level of the common femoral vein at the groin crease to the popliteal vein, but the technique is much less reliable for diagnosing calf vein thrombosis (Fig. 1.13). Approximately 40% of calf DVTs resolve spontaneously, 40% become organized and 20% propagate. Propagating DVT can be excluded by serial duplex scanning with an interval of 1 week.

I.v. contrast administered into the arm during CTPA can be used simultaneously to image for DVT. Such indirect CT venography (CTV) performs well in the detection of DVT, and is preferred to direct CTV where contrast is injected locally into a vein on the foot.

MR venography (MRV) is useful for examining the intracranial venous system, particularly in evaluating suspected dural venous sinus thrombosis, and for demonstrating venous thrombosis in the iliac vessels and abdomen. Non-contrast MRV requires a long acquisition time and provides only limited delineation of peripheral veins because of slow blood flow. Contrast-enhanced MRV uses i.v contrast administered into any vein, and newer contrast agents (e.g. gadofosveset trisodium) provide better spatial resolution.

MR direct thrombus imaging (MRDTI) uses the paramagnetic properties of methaemoglobin formed from oxidized haemoglobin within a thrombus to generate a signal. MRDTI provides images of the thrombus without relying on i.v contrast medium or blood flow to detect an intraluminal filling defect.

Venous reflux

Colour duplex has revolutionized the investigation of the lower limb venous system because it allows instantaneous visualization of blood flow and its direction (Figure 1.14). Thus, reflux at the saphenofemoral junction, saphenopopliteal junction and within the deep venous system, including the popliteal vein beneath the knee and the gastrocnemius veins, can be demonstrated noninvasively. Although a limited assessment of venous reflux can be undertaken using a pencil Doppler, compared with colour duplex the pencil Doppler misses ~12% of saphenofemoral and ~20% of saphenopopliteal junction reflux.

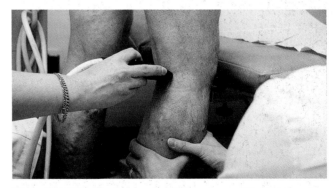

Figure 1.14 Colour duplex scanning of the saphenopopliteal junction. The calf muscles are manually compressed producing upward flow in the vein (top), which appears as a blue colour for flow towards the heart. Sudden release of the distal compression causes reflux, seen as a red colour, indicating flow away from the heart

Further reading

Burrill J, Dabbagh Z, Gollub F, *et al.* Multidetector computed tomographic angiography of the cardiovascular system. *Postgrad Med J* 2007;**83**:698–704.

McKenna M, Wolfson S, Kuller, L. The ratio of ankle and arm arterial pressure as an independent predictor of mortality. *Atherosclerosis* 1991;**87**:119–128.

Orbell JH, Smith A, Burnand KG, *et al.* Imaging of deep vein thrombosis. *Br J Surg* 2008;**95**:37–136.

Sheikh S, Gonzalez RG, Lev MH. Stroke CT angiography. In: Gonzalez RG, Hirsch JA, Koroshetz WJ *et al.*, eds. *Acute ischaemic stroke—imaging and intervention*. Springer, Berlin, 2006.

Stein PD, Hull RD. Multidetector computed tomography for the diagnosis of acute pulmonary embolism. *Curr Opin Pulm Med* 2007;**13**:384–388.

CHAPTER 2

Acute Limb Ischaemia

Timothy E Rowlands, Louise S Haine

OVERVIEW

- Acute limb ischaemia carries a high morbidity and mortality.
- Patients should receive intravenous heparin (and other resuscitative measures such as intravenous fluids and oxygen).
- Randomized trials have failed to show advantages between surgery and thrombolysis.
- Thrombolysis may help unmask lesions which permit further intervention, whether surgical or endovascular.
- A combined surgical and radiological multidisciplinary approach to patient care will give the best results.

Sudden loss of arterial blood supply to a limb is a surgical emergency. The effects of acute arterial occlusion depend on the state of collateral supply, and this is usually inadequate unless pre-existing occlusive disease is present. There is no single agreed definition of acute limb ischaemia, though suggested classifications exist (Table 2.1). Complete arterial ischaemia leads to tissue necrosis and the need for amputation within 6–12 h unless reperfusion occurs. Incomplete ischaemia is more common, and may be managed conservatively until a full assessment is undertaken and urgent treatment provided.

Clinical features

Many symptoms and signs of acute ischaemia are subtle. The infamous '6 Ps' (Table 2.2) are actually less commonly seen, with the exceptions of paralysis (unable to move the toes) and paraesthesia (loss of light touch over the back of the foot or hand). This reflects the often incomplete nature of the ischaemia.

The severity of the ischaemia at initial presentation determines the limb outcome. When arterial occlusion occurs there is usually intense vasospasm, during which the characteristic white appearance of the skin occurs. As this spasm decreases, a bluish mottled discoloration is seen due to the influx of deoxygenated blood into the skin, which will blanch. Calf pain and the suggestion of tense muscle compartments indicate muscle necrosis and impending irreversible ischaemia. Later, as coagulopathy occurs, there is a darker mottled appearance to the skin, which becomes fixed as irreversible tissue necrosis occurs. This final stage cannot be revascularized, and amputation becomes inevitable. These stages may be noted as the final events after a more insidious onset of acute ischaemia in a patient with pre-existing peripheral vascular disease (PVD), indicating a progressive deterioration in atherosclerotic vessels before a final occlusive thrombosis occurs.

Aetiology

Acute limb ischaemia is due to native arterial or bypass graft occlusion, and is generally embolic or thrombotic in origin (Table 2.3). In England and Wales, ~5000 patients present each year with acute limb ischaemia, and the associated mortality is ~20% with a limb loss rate of 30%. Mortality is higher in patients presenting with embolic causes, while limb loss is higher in those with thrombosis.

Embolic causes were historically the most common (now ~30–40%), due to valvular or ischaemic heart disease, with the passage of emboli from the ischaemic or fibrillating left atrium. Other causes include the passage of material from atherosclerotic plaques; this is cholesterol-rich instead of the platelet-rich material from the heart. The prognosis from this type of embolic episode is worse because embolectomy is generally less effective. Patients may present with digital emboli, the 'blue toe syndrome'.

Occasionally thrombus and atheromatous material from the subclavian artery can cause digital emboli in the hand, usually because of the presence of a dilated segment immediately distal to an area of compression due to a cervical rib. This can also be seen with other peripheral aneurysms (Figure 2.1).

Increased use of oral anticoagulants for atrial fibrillation has driven down the incidence of embolic phenomena, and the presentation of absolute ischaemia may actually be decreasing, perhaps because of statin usage and vessel collateralization. Trauma, or for example the loss of genicular vessels in knee replacement procedures, can however reduce these collaterals and the capacity to compensate for progressive large vessel stenosis in the presence of atherosclerosis.

ABC of Arterial & Venous Disease, 2nd edn. Edited by R. Donnelly and N. London.
© 2009 Blackwell Publishing Ltd. 9781405178891.

Table 2.1 SVS/ ISCVS guidelines for grading ischaemia (Rutherford *et al.*, 1997)

Class	Viability	Description
I	Viable	No sensorimotor impairment; Doppler signals audible
IIa	Marginally threatened	Mild sensory loss; inaudible Doppler signals
IIb	Immediately at risk	Significant sensory and motor loss; prompt treatment required to prevent limb loss
III	Irreversible	Complete sensory and motor loss with fixed skin mottling; attempts to restore circulation may be hazardous

Table 2.2 Symptoms and signs in acute limb ischaemia (the 6 Ps)

Symptoms/signs	Comments
Pain	May be absent with incomplete ischaemia
Pallor	Also seen in chronic ischaemia
Pulseless	As above
Paraesthesia	May progress to complete sensory and motor loss
Paralysis	Progression of paraesthesia
Perishing with cold	Unreliable as the limb may take on the ambient temperature

Table 2.3 Aetiology of acute ischaemia

Aetiology	Cause
Thrombosis	Atherosclerosis Bypass graft occlusion Prothrombotic conditions; protein C and S deficiency Popliteal aneurysm
Embolism	Atrial fibrillation Cardiac vegetations; rheumatic fever, i.v. drug users Mural thrombus; myocardial infarction Peripheral aneurysms Atheromatous plaque; blue toe syndrome Atrial myxoma
Rarities	Aortic dissection Trauma Intra-arterial drug injection Venous gangrene Saddle embolus Popliteal entrapment Cervical rib

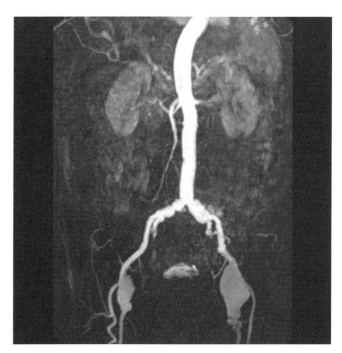

Figure 2.1 Magnetic resonance angiogram of a patient with bilateral femoral aneurysms: his abdominal aortic aneurysm was repaired several years before

Over the past 25 years there has been a gradual shift to thrombotic causes for most acute limb ischaemia (60%), with the increasing age of the population and increased incidence of PVD and diabetes (Figure 2.2). In those patients with bypass grafts, onset of acute ischaemia occurs in three broad phases: (1) early occlusion within the first month of surgery is usually due to technical failure and poor run-off; (2) medium-term failure at around 1 year is usually due to intimal hyperplasia or new stenoses within a vein graft; and (3) late failure is generally due to progressive PVD and continued smoking.

Popliteal aneurysms are particularly difficult to treat. Acute thrombosis is associated with a high risk of limb loss due to occlusion of the popliteal artery and the propagation of thrombus into the crural vessels of the foot. Treatment is aimed at clearing the thrombus from these distal vessels, with exclusion bypass of the aneurysm itself. The detection of a popliteal aneurysm should prompt clinical examination of the other side, since bilateral disease is common (Figure 2.3).

Many other factors predispose to the development of *in situ* thrombosis, including dehydration, the presence of malignancy, hyperviscosity and prothrombotic syndromes. These latter syndromes should be considered in younger patients without vascular risk factors, along with anatomical rarities such as popliteal entrapment.

Management

General measures

Acute ischaemia is a condition where lack of prompt assessment by a vascular specialist will have an adverse effect on outcome. A delay

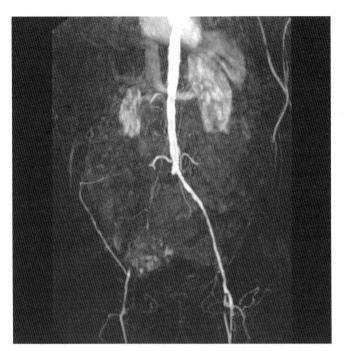

Figure 2.2 Magnetic resonance angiogram from a patient with previous claudication presenting with thrombosis of the right common and external iliac arteries: ischaemia was incomplete due to extensive collateralization

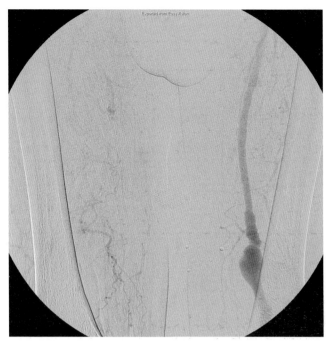

Figure 2.3 Arteriogram demonstrating incidental asymptomatic left popliteal aneurysm during the presentation of acute right limb ischaemia from a thrombosed right popliteal aneurysm: the right-sided aneurysm is not seen due to loss of run-off

of 6 h can make the difference between successful limb salvage and amputation or death.

Initial treatment should include i.v fluids, and i.v heparin unless absolutely contraindicated. The heparin is to limit the damage by further propagation of thrombus, but may also improve outcomes. The duration of the current symptoms and a previous history of intermittent claudication should be carefully noted in the history.

A key question in the initial management is the need for immediate vascular imaging such as angiography (Figure 2.4). A completely ischaemic limb should be explored in the operating theatre without delay, especially if the clinical picture suggests a likelihood of embolus (a rapid deterioration in the limb with normal pulses in the contralateral limb often indicates an embolic cause). More frequently though, with lesser degrees of ischaemia, there is time for pre-operative angiography. This allows other timely therapeutic options to be considered, including thrombolysis, angioplasty, stenting or bypass.

A completely non-viable limb needs to be recognized, as revascularization would be inappropriate and hazardous. Amputation or even terminal care in the moribund patient should be considered early.

Surgery

Balloon embolectomy remains the standard initial operative treatment of an embolus. The technique can be performed quickly under local anaesthetic, without the need for pre-operative angiography which may cause unnecessary delay. Following embolectomy, angiography can be performed in the operating theatre to check the result. If the initial procedure is unsatisfactory, further

surgical options might include immediate popliteal exposure, bypass or on-table thrombolysis.

This is an uncommon scenario, and few patients thankfully need such immediate intervention, but it takes considerable experience to be able to decide which patients can and cannot wait for specialist timely intervention.

Surgery plays a major role in non-embolic causes of acute limb ischaemia, though with a wider series of options. In cases of trauma

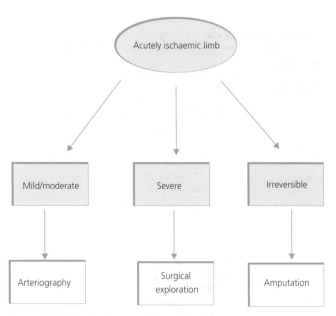

Figure 2.4 Initial triage in acute ischaemia

Table 2.4 Contraindications to thrombolysis

Pregnancy
Stroke within 2 months
Vascular surgery within 2 weeks
Trauma within 2 weeks
Transient ischaemic attack within 2 weeks
Previous gastrointestinal tract bleeding
Craniotomy in previous 2 months
Active bleeding
Known severe bleeding tendency
Intracerebral arteriovenous malformation/tumour/aneurysm
Recent eye surgery

such as supracondylar fracture of the elbow or posterior dislocation of the knee, angiography may direct the relative involvement of surgical bypass or endovascular intervention. Thrombosis in a patient with pre-existing disease is less likely to present as absolute ischaemia, hence pre-operative angiography is feasible and introduces many other therapeutic options, including thrombolysis.

Thrombolysis

Initial results with systemic administration of thrombolytic agents (using protocols devised for acute myocardial infarction) were poor, but refinement of techniques has since occurred. Intra-arterial, catheter-directed infusion of thrombolytics (e.g. tissue plasminogen activator) is currently the best way of achieving revascularization; dosage regimes via the catheter vary depending on local expertise. Thrombolysis is generally less invasive, and can open small vessels as well as larger ones, improving patency. Thrombolysis is also effective at unmasking the arterial lesions which triggered *in situ* thrombosis, allowing subsequent angioplasty, stenting or bypass.

There are many potential complications, not least because patients are usually elderly with concurrent cardiovascular co-morbidities. There is potentially a higher risk of ongoing limb ischaemia, and of haemorrhagic complications, including stroke, than from surgery. The higher risk of complications from thrombolysis must be balanced against the risks of surgery in each patient. There are many relative contraindications, though perhaps the only absolute contraindication is active internal bleeding. Local policy defines these contraindications (Table 2.4).

Several randomized trials have been performed, with no overall difference in limb salvage or death between initial surgery and initial thrombolysis. Universal recommendations for initial treatment (either surgery or thrombolysis) cannot be advocated on current evidence. Both have distinct roles to play, and emphasize the close collaboration required locally between surgeons and interventional radiologists to achieve the best outcome for the patient.

The sequelae of revascularization

Ischaemia–reperfusion

Reintroducing the blood supply to a previously ischaemic tissue can cause further damage over and above that of the ischaemia alone. This is termed ischaemia–reperfusion injury and is seen in a variety of other clinical settings, such as myocardial infarction and transplantation. This is a complex process associated with the delivery and generation of oxygen free radicals within ischaemic tissue, with neutrophil activation. The action of neutrophils on the vascular endothelium is ultimately to promote oedema and cell death on a wide scale. The net effect is to damage tissue locally, and also at remote sites, via the excessive production of inflammatory mediators.

Compartment syndrome occurs locally in the limb due to oedema within the individual muscle compartments. Muscle dysfunction occurs, and, unless the raised interstitial pressure within all the compartments is relieved by fasciotomy, the muscle becomes non-viable and toxic. The patient will usually complain of pain, with exquisite tenderness on squeezing the calf or passive dorsiflexion of the foot. Pedal pulses may still be present. Debate on the value of compartment pressure measurement is usually irrelevant; emergency fasciotomy wounds can be closed or skin-grafted later. There is often a degree of oedema seen permanently in the revascularized limb as a consequence of ischaemia–reperfusion injury.

Remote organ dysfunction and the systemic inflammatory response syndrome (SIRS) are frequently observed. Metabolic acidosis and hyperkalaemia with rhabdomyolysis from muscle death may lead to acute tubular necrosis and significant risk of acute renal failure. Myocardial depression can occur, with shock and infarction, and acute respiratory distress. It is these side effects that contribute significantly to the high mortality of acute limb ischaemia.

Chronic limb pain

Patients with successful revascularization frequently complain of limb pain afterwards. This is probably due to nerve injury from the original ischaemic insult. Treatment may involve different combination drug treatments such as opiates, gabapentin and antidepressants; non-steroidal drugs are often of little use. Other treatments include sympathectomy, or the use of spinal cord stimulators, under specialist guidance.

New developments

The attractive prospect of being able to remove thrombus rapidly without the attendant risks of thrombolytic therapy or general anaesthesia has helped to drive the development and implementation of new techniques. Aspiration thrombectomy can be performed by the interventionalist and is a useful technique to remove small quantities of thrombus.

Mechanical thrombectomy involves breaking up existing thrombus, and aspirating it. Thrombus is broken up from solid material into particulate matter either by means of a high-speed rotating brush or basket (Cragg brush), or by creation of vortices at the catheter tip which suck up and disperse thrombus using the Venturi effect (Angiojet). Haemolysis and blood loss do occur, particularly with prolonged use. Evidence for these devices is currently lacking, but with further refinements to the technique and equipment they may offer future potential.

Further reading

Blaisdell FW, Steele M, Allen RF. Management of acute lower limb ischaemia due to embolism and thrombosis. *Surgery* 1978;**84**:822–834.

Campbell WB. Non-intervention and palliative care in vascular patients. *Br J Surg* 2000;**87**:1601–1602.

Campbell WB, Ridler BMF, Symanska TH, on behalf of the Vascular Surgical Society of Great Britain and Ireland. Current management of acute leg ischaemia: results of an audit by the Vascular Surgical Society of Great Britain and Ireland. *Br J Surg* 1998;**85**:1498–1503.

Rutherford RB, Baker JD, Ernst C *et al.* Recommended standards for reports dealing with lower extremity ischaemia: revised version. *J Vasc Surg* 1997;**26**:517–538.

The STILE Investigators. Results of a prospective randomized trial evaluating surgery versus thrombolysis for ischaemia of the lower extremity. *Ann Surg* 1994;**220**:251–268.

CHAPTER 3

Chronic Lower Limb Ischaemia

Martin JS Dennis, William D Adair, Amman Bolia

OVERVIEW

- The diagnosis of peripheral arterial disease is based mainly on the history.
- Intermittent claudication is a marker for widespread atherosclerosis. The risk to limb is low, the risk to life is high.
- In patients with intermittent claudication, the primary role of the doctor is to address and correct risk factors for atherosclerosis.
- Patients with critical ischaemia require urgent referral to a vascular surgeon who, in addition to correcting risk factors, will revascularize the leg.
- The minority of patients with intermittent claudication will benefit from intervention, whereas the majority of patients with critical ischaemia require angioplasty and/or bypass surgery.
- Remember that in chronic critical limb ischaemia the foot may be paradoxically pink—the so-called 'sunset foot'.

Introduction

This chapter covers the clinical aspects of chronic lower limb ischaemia. By convention, the symptoms or signs of leg ischaemia must have been present for 2 weeks to be correctly described as chronic. There are two important points to bear in mind when assessing patients with chronic leg ischaemia:

1. Always remember that the affected leg is part of a patient who must be assessed as a whole, both medically and in their family and social setting.
2. PVD can be asymptomatic at one end of the scale, or at the other end of the scale lead to critical ischaemia with limb loss (Figure 3.1).

Why do patients get chronic lower limb ischaemia?

The majority of cases will be due to atherosclerosis. This is the predominant disease in most developed countries and, if present

in the legs, will also have affected the coronary and cerebral arteries. Since the prevalence of atherosclerosis increases with age, most patients will be over 55. It is a mistake, however, to assume that a younger patient cannot have PVD. A 30 or 40 year old can present with premature atherosclerosis caused by diabetes, familial hyperlipidaemia or smoking. The other pathologies to keep in mind are those which cause acute limb ischaemia but whose effects persist and become chronic. These are arterial embolism, thrombosis of limb aneurysms and arterial dissection.

Lower limb arterial anatomy

It is useful to review this because atherosclerosis predictably affects certain sites in the limb and this causes characteristic symptoms (Figure 3.2). Atheroma tends to form where arteries are fixed posteriorly by branching.

What history will a patient with chronic leg ischaemia give?

The most common symptoms are intermittent claudication (IC)—pain in the calf muscles, induced by exercise and relieved by rest. Less commonly the thigh and buttock are affected. The muscle pain results from anaerobic muscle metabolism during exercise and is caused by an obstruction to arterial blood flow due to one of the causes listed above.

IC is rare in patients under 55 years of age but affects at least 5% of those aged 55–74. At younger ages, the prevalence of IC is almost twice as high in men as women, but the gender difference narrows in older patients.

As the ABPI drops with progressively worsening PVD so the claudication distance reduces, and eventually perfusion to the foot is so compromised that the patient complains of rest pain. Rest pain is pain in the foot at night, often relieved by hanging the leg out of bed. This manoeuvre adds the assistance of gravity to the feeble foot perfusion. Indeed, some patients are afraid to go to bed, and sleep in a chair all night. If not improved by vascular intervention, the circulation may continue to deteriorate, resulting in ulceration or gangrene. If these are present for >2 weeks, the pain requires analgesia and if the measured arterial pressure at the ankle is

ABC of Arterial & Venous Disease, 2nd edn. Edited by R. Donnelly and N. London.
© 2009 Blackwell Publishing Ltd. 9781405178891.

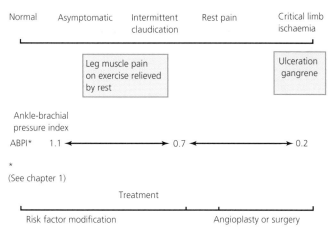

Figure 3.1 The spectrum of lower limb vascular disease

<50 mmHg then by definition the patient has critical limb isch-aemia (CLI). Although IC is common, CLI is rare, with an esti-mated incidence of only 500–1000 per million per year.

What are the important differential diagnoses?

1. Nerve root compression—tends to be a sharp shooting pain radiating down the back of the leg and often relieved by adjust-ing posture rather than rest. Pain may come on when sitting or standing, not with exercise.
2. Spinal stenosis—although the patient with spinal stenosis may complain of calf, thigh and/or buttock pain on exercise, the fol-lowing symptoms point to 'spinal' rather than vascular claudica-tion. The pain may be described as coming 'down the back of the leg' and may be associated with back pain, numbness, tin-gling or 'shooting pains'. In 90% of cases prolonged standing brings on the pain. The patient may note weakness, heaviness or numbness of the leg on exercise and may adopt a 'simian stance' in which they stand or walk in a partly flexed position. Many patients will lean against a wall or sit down when they have to stop walking in order to achieve spinal flexion and relieve their pain.
3. Leg symptoms on exercise can be a diagnostic challenge as in the elderly patient several conditions can co-exist, e.g. lumbo sacral spine disease and PVD.

Examination of the patient with PVD

Always examine the whole arterial tree.

LOOK carefully for ulcers between the toes and under the heels. Hair loss is a useful physical sign.

FEEL for pulses. Femoral pulses are best felt with the legs almost straight, a little abducted and the feet externally rotated. Popliteal pulses are palpated behind the upper tibia with the knee extended. Skin temperature is an unreliable finding in CLI, but very impor-tant in acute limb ischaemia. The usual pattern of pulses in a patient with calf claudication will be a good femoral pulse, absent popliteal and pedal pulses, but a healthy foot. If the disease affects the iliac arteries, the symptoms will usually be thigh and buttock claudication, perhaps with impotence. The femoral pulse will be

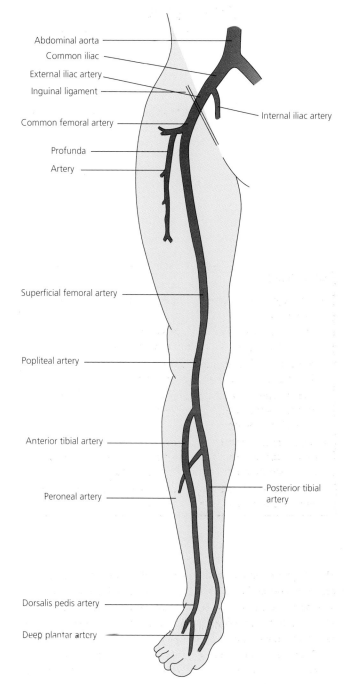

Figure 3.2 Leg arterial anatomy

reduced or absent on that side. In patients with a proximal stenosis it is possible to have palpable pedal pulses at rest that disappear on exercise. Thus the presence of pedal pulses does not exclude a diagnosis of claudication.

CHECK for capillary refill time (normal is <3 s) and in a patient with rest pain perform Buerger's test. In a limb with CLI the skin vessels may be maximally dilated, producing a 'sunset' foot which appears pink and even warm. However, when the foot is elevated, the severity of the ischaemia is revealed, with severe pallor and venous guttering (Figure 3.3). Misdiagnosing the sunset foot of CLI as cellulitis is a potential pitfall for the unwary.

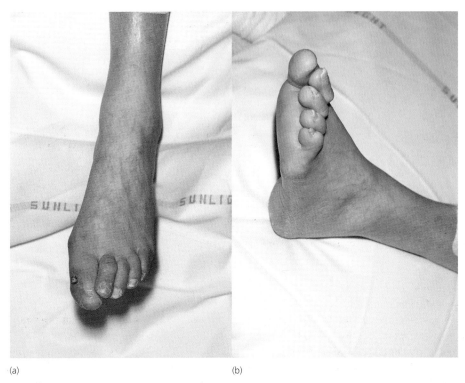

(a)   (b)

Figure 3.3 (a) A positive Buerger's test in critical limb ischaemia, (b) a sunset foot when dependent, blanching when elevated

Investigations

The vascular status of the lower limb at rest is best assessed by listening to pedal signals from a hand-held pencil Doppler or by measurement of the ABPI. The best way to assess whether the arterial supply to the lower limb is impaired on exercise is a walk test. If indicated, the arterial tree is imaged non-invasively with colour duplex ultrasound scanning and occasionally MRA or CTA. This allows selection of an appropriate puncture site for digital subtraction angiography (DSA) and endovascular intervention.

Treatment of PVD

Claudication

The prognosis for patients with IC is poor. They have a mortality of 12% a year—66% die from heart disease and 10% due to strokes

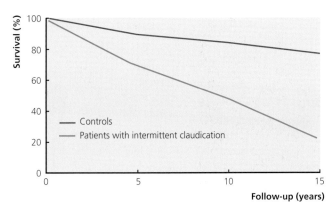

Figure 3.4 Survival in patients with intermittent claudication (IC) compared with age-matched healthy controls

(Figure 3.4). The prognosis for their affected leg is very good (Figure 3.5). Reduced ABPI is a proven predictor of premature cardiovascular death, irrespective of whether the patient is complaining of IC symptoms. The primary role of the doctor is to engage with the patient to address and correct the risk factors for atherosclerosis. Although historically a large number of drugs have been prescribed to treat IC, the evidence behind their use is poor. More recently, cilostazol, a phosphodiesterase inhibitor, has been used to treat IC. There is some evidence of benefit. The precise role of cilostazol remains to be defined, but it may be worth trying in patients who do not improve at all after 6 months of adherence to best medical treatment.

Should claudicants ever have interventional treatment?

Only a minority of patients with IC will need angioplasty or surgery. This is because most will get better and live longer with exercise and risk factor modification. Invasive treatment (angioplasty or surgery) becomes appropriate with failure to respond to conservative measures and if PVD is severely affecting lifestyle. Once all risk factors have been corrected, angioplasty is useful in iliac and superficial femoral artery disease. On the very rare occasions that surgery is performed, it is most commonly because of failed iliac or superficial femoral artery angioplasty.

Critical limb ischaemia

The survival of patients with CLI is very poor. Twenty percent will die within a year, and the 5-year mortality is >50%. This is due to their advanced co-existent cardiac and cerebrovascular arterial disease. The treatment goal is **limb salvage**. This is because major limb amputation is a terrible trauma for the patient, not cost-effective and usually results in a wheelchair existence and

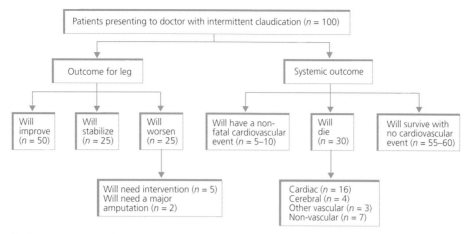

Figure 3.5 Intermittent claudication—prognosis for patients and their legs. From Burns *et al.* (2003)

housing problems. Limb salvage is achieved by restoring adequate arterial foot perfusion. In suitably skilled vascular units, the first-line treatment for CLI is percutaneous angioplasty under local anaesthetic. There are two techniques for angioplasty—luminal and subintimal (Figure 3.6).

Single superficial femoral artery (SFA) or popliteal stenosis <3 cm in length are ideally treated by luminal angioplasty, whilst long (<5 cm) stenoses or occlusions, particularly in the presence of heavy calcification, are best treated by subintimal angioplasty (Figure 3.7).

High rates of limb salvage are achieved by subintimal angioplasty. The technique, although demanding a high radiological skill level, is attractive due to the added benefits of reduced patient morbidity and mortality, short hospital stay and cost-effectiveness. Additionally the option remains for repeat intervention—either radiological or surgical. Angioplasty of the iliac segment is some-times combined with deployment of an endovascular stent (Figure 3.8).

If angioplasty is unsuccessful, then bypass grafting should be considered. This is nearly always done using the patient's own saphenous or arm vein as the bypass conduit. The results of bypass grafting for CLI can be excellent, with 5-year limb salvage rates as high as 80%. There may be occasions when a reasonably fit patient has lost so much tissue in the foot that any attempt to save it is futile. Similarly, patients who have developed fixed flexion contractions of the knee and the hip may be best managed by primary amputation. If the general condition of the patient is so poor and the chances of survival limited by co-morbidity, it may be appropriate simply to make the patient comfortable. These decisions are best made in consultation with the patient, relatives and the rehabilitation team looking after the patient.

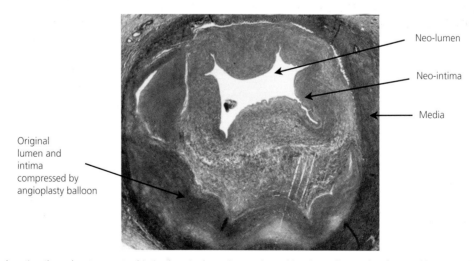

Figure 3.6 Histological section through artery post-subintimal angioplasty. A new channel has been dissected and opened between the intima and the media. In conventional angioplasty, recannalization is confined to the arterial lumen. Courtesy of Dr Tor Florenes, Aker University Hospital, Oslo, Norway

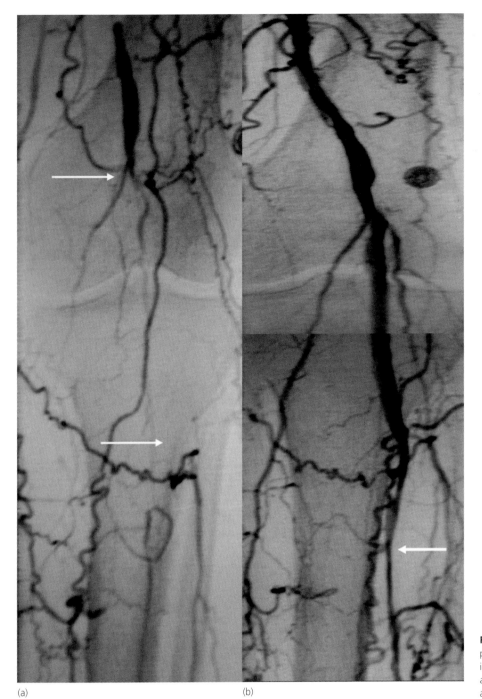

Figure 3.7 Angiogram (a) showing a popliteal occlusion (between arrows). Run-off is via collaterals only. Following subintimal angioplasty (b) the popliteal and peroneal arteries (arrow) have been recannalized

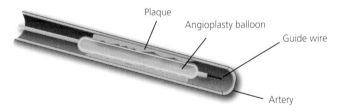

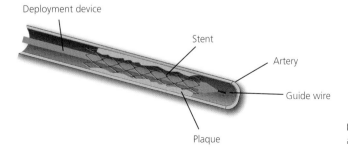

Figure 3.8 Techniques for endovascular recannalization include balloon angioplasty with or without a metal stent

Further reading

Burns P, Gough S, Bradbury AW. Management of peripheral arterial disease in primary care. *BMJ* 2003;**326**:584–588.

Cassar K. Intermittent claudication. *BMJ* 2006;**333**:1002–1005.

Norgren L, Hiatt WR, Dormandy JA *et al*; TASC II Working Group. Inter-society consensus for the management of peripheral arterial disease (TASC II). *Eur J Vasc Endovasc Surg* 2007;**33**(Suppl.)S5–S67.

Rowlands TE, Donnelly R. Medical therapy for intermittent claudication. *Eur J Vasc Endovasc Surg* 2007;**34**:314–321.

Shearman CP. Management of intermittent claudication. *Br J Surg* 2002;**89**:529–531.

CHAPTER 4

Cerebrovascular Disease

Christopher I Price, Gary A Ford

OVERVIEW

- Stroke and transient ischaemic attack are common medical emergencies.
- Effective care requires rapid access to a specialist multidisciplinary team.
- Thrombolysis for stroke under specialist supervision reduces disability.
- Treatment and rehabilitation on a stroke unit reduces death, disability, complications and costs.
- Modifiable risk factors are common and should be assessed systematically.

Stroke and transient ischaemic attack (TIA) require rapid assessment and multidisciplinary management in order to reduce mortality, long-term disability and costs to society (Box 4.1). Each year in the UK there are 110 000 new cases of stroke, contributing 11% to national mortality statistics. There are 300 000 people living with the consequences of stroke, including 100 000 who require daily assistance with personal care.

Box 4.1 Costs associated with stroke per year (National Audit Office 2005)

- £2.8 billion   direct costs (healthcare)
- £1.8 billion   indirect costs (loss of earnings, benefits claimed)
- £2.4 billion   'informal' care costs (care provided free by families)
- £7.0 billion   total costs

TIA has a lifetime prevalence of 5 per 1000 population, and although by definition there is no initial permanent neurological deficit, 17% of patients will suffer a stroke during the next 3 months. The risk for some patients is as high as 1 in 3 during the week after

ABC of Arterial & Venous Disease, 2nd edn. Edited by R. Donnelly and N. London.
© 2009 Blackwell Publishing Ltd. 9781405178891.

their TIA symptoms. Therefore, both stroke and TIA should be referred immediately for specialist inpatient or outpatient assessment in order to institute measures that reduce the risk of subsequent disability and death.

Aetiology

TIAs and 85% of strokes are due to atherothrombotic occlusion of a cerebral artery or cardioembolism. Neurons are extremely oxygen dependent, and an irreversible process of cell death begins if perfusion is not quickly restored. Haemorrhage accounts for 15% of strokes, mainly from primary intracerebral haemorrhage due to small vessel lipohyalinosis. This causes tissue damage through compression and reactive vasospasm. However, one-third of patients may have an underlying tumour, aneurysm or arteriovenous malformation, so further investigations should be considered for those surviving without major disability.

Stroke predominantly occurs in older people at an average age of 74 years, but 15% are under the age of 60 years (Table 4.1). For younger patients it is important to consider mechanisms other than atheroma for ischaemic stroke, such as carotid dissection, patent foramen ovale, thrombophilia and uncommon genetic disorders such as CADASIL or Fabry's disease. However, no definitive cause is identified in one-third of patients despite investigations.

Clinical assessment

Stroke and TIA are the initial clinical diagnoses suspected when there has been an acute-onset focal neurological deficit with a likely vascular origin. The typical duration of TIA is <20 min, although for practical and demographic purposes the World Health Organization (WHO) definition permits symptoms to persist up to 24 h. However, unless there has been complete recovery at the time of medical review and the immediate risk of stroke is low, the patient should be admitted for neurological monitoring and urgent assessment.

Many conditions can present in a similar way to stroke (Table 4.2). Particular care should be taken when there is a global disturbance of consciousness (Glasgow Coma Score (GCS) <8), as this hinders identification of precise neurological deficits and increases

Table 4.1 Important risk factors for ischaemic stroke and TIA

	Clinical note	Assessment	First-line management
Atherothrombotic			
Hypertension	50% patients have systolic BP > 160 mmHg at presentation	<140/85 is secondary prevention target (with diabetes BP target <130/80)	BP-lowering drugs and lifestyle advice
Diabetes mellitus	40% patients have moderate hyperglycaemia at presentation	Diagnose if fasting glucose >6.1 mmol/l	Diet and glucose-lowering drugs
Hypercholesterolaemia	Check within 24 h of event	Treat if total cholesterol >3.5 mmol/l	Statin
Smoking	Doubles the risk of stroke recurrence	Document pack years	Refer to smoking cessation service
Carotid artery stenosis	Adhere to local protocol for carotid ultrasound	Considering treating symptomatic side stenosis of 70–99%	Carotid endarterectomy
Carotid dissection	Neck pain and Horner's syndrome 30% of younger ischaemic stroke	CT or MR angiography of neck vessels	Anticoagulation or antiplatelet drugs for 3–6 months
Thrombophilia	Reserve for younger patients without vascular risk factors	Thrombophilia screen	Anticoagulation depending upon result, individual risk and choice
Cardioembolism			
Atrial fibrillation	Consider 24 h ECG if recurrent events	ECG	Long-term anticoagulation
Recent MI	Highest risk is anterior MI < 4 weeks	ECG. Transthoracic echocardiogram	Anticoagulation for 3–6 months
Left ventricular aneurysm	ECG with ST elevation	Transthoracic echocardiogram	Long-term anticoagulation
Patent foramen ovale	Younger patients without vascular risk factors	Transoesophageal echocardiogram	Consider closure or anticoagulation if aneurismal atrial septal defect and/or previous events

MI = myocardial infarction.

the probability of an alternative mechanism for any focal signs. It may be necessary to obtain urgently a witness account of events, past medical history, laboratory results and radiological assessment in order to exclude a condition which requires specific emergency treatment, e.g. dextrose for hypoglycaemia.

After making an initial diagnosis of stroke, it is necessary to determine the clinical stroke subtype in order to describe the severity and pattern of the neurological deficit, estimate prognosis and facilitate clinical audit. The clinical effects of stroke depend upon the vascular territory of the brain involved. The Oxfordshire Community Stroke Project classification correlates clinical signs with cerebral vascular territory, which is divided into anterior (carotid) and posterior (vertebrobasilar) circulations (Table 4.3).

Radiological assessment

Rapid CT scanning is the most appropriate initial brain imaging for most cases, as this will exclude haemorrhage even if signs of

Table 4.2 Common stroke mimics

Cause	Useful features
Seizures	Previous episodes. Low GCS at presentation for the size of focal deficit
Syncope (and cerebral hypoperfusion)	Witnessed loss of consciousness. Features improve with volume expansion
Sepsis (especially after previous stroke)	Fluctuating neurological features. Raised CRP. Insidious onset
Somatization	Inconsistent signs. Low vascular risk. History of other unexplained symptoms
Space-occupying lesion	Subacute onset. Previous primary tumour. Papilloedema
Sugar (hypoglycaemia and hyperglycaemia)	Disorientated/drowsy with minimal weakness. Medication
Subdural (including unwitnessed head trauma)	Fluctuating signs. Disorientated/drowsy. Frequent faller. No sepsis.
Single nerve injury (including Bell's palsy)	Sensorimotor deficit in isolated nerve. Dermatomal and lower motor features
Severe migraine (without headache)	Previous episodes of neurological migraine. Progressive symptoms
Sclerosis (demyelination)	Previous episodes in different vascular territories. Subacute onset.

CRP = C-reactive protein; GCS = Glasgow Coma Score.

Table 4.3 Clinical classification of stroke and prognosis using the Oxfordshire Community Stroke Project categories

Clinical features on examination:

1. Unilateral weakness/sensory deficit of face?
2. Unilateral weakness/sensory deficit of arm/hand?
3. Unilateral weakness/sensory deficit of leg/foot?
4. Dysphasia? (note cerebral dominance)
5. Visuospatial disorder?
6. Homonymous hemianopia?
7. Brainstem/cerebellar signs (ataxia/diplopia)?

Subgroup	Feature combinations	Lesion site	Cortical deficit	Prognosis at 6 months	
				% Dead	% Dependent
LACS	1 + 2 2 + 3 1 + 2 + 3	Internal capsule	No	11	28
PACS	Any one of 1–5 alone 1 ± 2 ± 3 plus only one of 4, 5 or 6	Cortex (branch of middle cerebral artery)	Yes (only one)	16	29
TACS	Any two of 4, 5 and 6 Usually accompanied by 1 + 2 + 3	Cortex (middle cerebral artery)	Yes (more than one)	60	36
POCS	6 alone 7 alone 6 + 7	Brainstem and/or cerebellum and/or occipital cortex hemianopia/cortical blindness (basilar or posterior cerebral artery)	None or only	19	19

LACS = lacunar anterior circulation stroke; PACS = partial anterior circulation stroke; POCS = posterior circulation stroke; TACS = total anterior circulation stroke.

infarction are not present. It should be performed within 24 h of symptom onset, although economic analysis has demonstrated that the most efficient system is for all patients to receive imaging on admission. The next available scan slot should be requested for patients who are unconscious, taking anticoagulants, eligible for thrombolytic therapy, exhibiting unexpected deterioration or if there is any suggestion of head injury. When there is uncertainty about diagnosis, magnetic resonance imaging (MRI) with diffusion-weighted imaging (DWI) is very useful as it is highly specific for cerebral ischaemia within the previous 7–10 days.

Advanced CT or MRI with angiography and perfusion imaging is increasingly being used to identify patients most suitable for thrombolytic therapy (Figures 4.1–4.3).

Emergency management

The public should be encouraged to call 999 if they have reason to believe that they are suffering from a possible stroke or 'brain attack'. To promote the accurate recognition of stroke by emergency services, simple screening tools are available for use by the public and paramedics (Face Arm Speech Test; Figure 4.4) and emergency department staff (ROSIER score; Figure 4.5). Direct referral can then be made to the local stroke service according to an agreed ambulance protocol.

During acute ischaemic stroke, ~1.9 million neurons die per minute. Recombinant tissue plasminogen activator (alteplase) is a National Institute for Health and Clinical Excellence (NICE)-

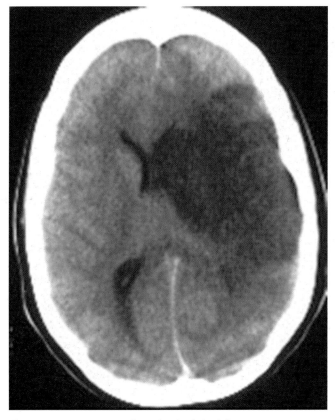

Figure 4.1 CT appearance of anterior circulation infarct

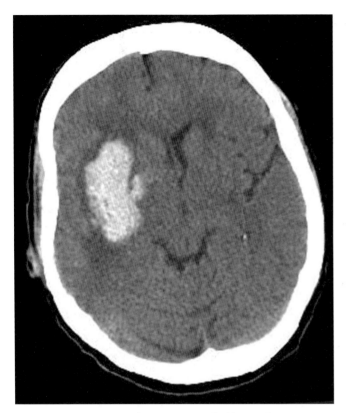

Figure 4.2 CT appearance of primary intracerebral haemorrhage

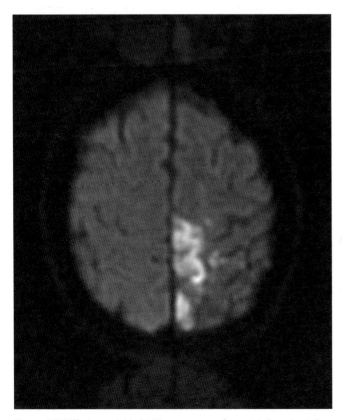

Figure 4.3 Diffusion-weighted MRI appearance of recent ischaemic stroke

SPINAL BOARD		CERVICAL COLLAR
R.E.D.		ORTHO. STRETCHER
VACUUM MAT		OTHER

11.STROKE (FACE ARM SPEECH TEST)		
SPEECH IMPAIRMENT	YES ☑	NO ☐
FACIAL PALSY	YES ☑	NO ☐
AFFECTED SIDE	L ☑	R ☐
ARM WEAKNESS?	YES ☑	NO ☐
AFFECTED SIDE	L ☑	R ☐

| **12.CANNULATION** | | |
| SIZE | 14g ☐ | 16g ☐ | 18g ☐ |

Figure 4.4 The FAST on an ambulance report form

Assessment   Date ☐☐☐☐☐☐   Time ☐☐☐☐

Symptom onset Date ☐☐☐☐☐☐   Time ☐☐☐☐

GCS E=☐ M=☐ V=☐   BP ☐☐   *BM ☐

*IF BM<3.5mmol/L treat urgently and reassess once blood glucose normal

Has there been loss of consciousness or syncope?   Y(−1)☐   N(0)☐

Has there been seizure activity?   Y(−1)☐   N(0)☐

Is there a <u>NEW ACUTE</u> onset (or on awakening from sleep)

I.   Asymmetric facial weakness   Y(+1)☐   N(0)☐

II.   Asymmetric arm weakness   Y(+1)☐   N(0)☐

III. Asymmetric leg weakness   Y(+1)☐   N(0)☐

IV.   Speech disturbance   Y(+1)☐   N(0)☐

V.   Visual field defect   Y(+1)☐   N(0)☐

*Total Score _____ (−2 to +5)

Provision diagnosis

☐ Stoke   ☐ Non-stroke (specify) _____

*Stroke is unlikely but not completely excluded if total scores are ⩽ 0.

Figure 4.5 The ROSIER score

recommended therapy which reduces disability by restoring perfusion to acutely ischaemic areas. It must be administered in <3 h according to strict criteria under the supervision of a physician with expertise in stroke assessment (Box 4.2). For every seven stroke patients treated, one will avoid death or long-term disability. The reduction in infarct size is offset by an increased risk of intracranial haemorrhage, which is fatal in 2–3% of cases. Overall, 1 patient in 3 gains some functional improvement from thrombolytic therapy whereas 1 in 33 is harmed. Stroke services must be able to monitor patients so that the risk of symptomatic haemorrhage is minimized and react rapidly if there is a neurological deterioration.

Box 4.2 **Main eligibility criteria for thrombolysis of acute ischaemic stroke**

- Administration <3 h since symptom onset
- No haemorrhage on CT scan
- No extensive signs of early ischaemia on CT scan
- National Institute of Health Stroke Score 5–24
- Independently mobile prior to stroke
- No seizure since stroke onset
- Blood pressure <185/110 mmHg
- No history of intracranial haemorrhage
- No history of stroke in <3 months
- No surgery or gastrointestinal bleeding <3 weeks
- No other recent significant haemorrhage
- No hypoglycaemia or severe hyperglycaemia (blood glucose 2.7–22 mmol/l)
- International normalized ratio (INR) <1.4 if taking warfarin
- Platelet count >100

Patients with primary intracerebal haemorrhage do not routinely benefit from surgical intervention, although individual cases should be discussed with the local neurosurgical service (Table 4.4). Clinical trials so far have not shown any immediate advantage from neuroprotective agents, glucose lowering or blood pressure modification in acute haemorrhagic or ischaemic stroke.

Stroke unit care

All stroke patients should be admitted to an Acute Stroke Unit as soon as possible. It has been clearly demonstrated that rapid admission of patients to a geographically defined stroke unit reduces mortality, disability and length of inpatient stay. The number needed to treat (NNT) in organized stroke care is only 16 before achieving a significantly better outcome for 1 patient. This treatment effect is spread across the interventions provided by the multidisciplinary team during the whole admission. Units also provide palliative care for a small number of patients because of stroke severity and pre-existing co-morbidities. For this group, specialist

assessment ensures that potentially treatable conditions have been excluded, such as seizures and metabolic disturbance.

Box 4.3 **Summary of interventions for acute stroke**

- Assess for thrombolysis eligibility
- Request CT brain scan (consider whether urgent scan indicated)
- Administer 300 mg aspirin by mouth, rectum or nasogastric tube if no haemorrhage on CT
- Avoid heparin unless known high risk for pulmonary embolism (consider prophylaxis)
- Routine bloods (including lipids, glucose and inflammatory markers)
- Record ECG
- Assess swallow safety, and modify diet accordingly
- Assess pressure sore risk
- Physiological monitoring of temperature, heart rate, blood pressure, oxygen saturation
- Re-assess patients with pyrexia and undertake active cooling
- Early mobilization
- Provide patient and carers with information on diagnosis and prognosis

Swallowing is impaired following stroke in ~50% of patients, although many can manage safe oral intake of a modified diet under nursing supervision with speech therapy guidance. Temporary nasogastric feeding should be started within 24–48 h of stroke in conscious patients who cannot demonstrate safe swallowing. There is no significant survival advantage from insertion of a percutaneous endoscopic gastrostomy (PEG) tube earlier than 1 month, as swallowing will often improve quickly for many patients, whilst those with severe swallowing problems have a high early mortality related to the underlying stroke severity (Box 4.3).

Rehabilitation after stroke

Patients should undergo repeated multidisciplinary assessment of their individual needs, co-ordinated by a weekly team meeting to

Table 4.4 Indications for neuroscience consultation

Scenario	Possible intervention
Suspected basilar artery thrombosis <24 h	Intra-arterial thrombolysis
Superficial primary intracerebral haemorrhage with further neurological deterioration	Surgical evacuation if early and patient conscious
Haemorrhage with suspected underlying aneurysm	Angiography and clipping or radiological coiling. Hydrocephalus treatment
Conscious level deterioration following posterior fossa haematoma	Surgical evacuation and hydrocephalus treatment
Conscious level deterioration following large MCA infarct (malignant MCA infarction due to oedema)	Decompressive craniectomy if early and no significant co-morbidities

MCA = middle cerebral artery.

document updated rehabilitation goals and review discharge arrangements. Early mobilization is very important, as it reduces risk of DVT and pressure sores, minimizes muscular atrophy and spasticity, prevents abnormal posture development and provides patients with tactile and cognitive stimulation. There is increasing evidence that rehabilitation programmes which contain repetitive task-orientated movements produce quicker and greater improvements in motor recovery (Box 4.4).

Box 4.4 **Complications during rehabilitation**

- Pain
- Malnutrition
- Incontinence
- Pressure sores
- Falls
- Spasticity
- Isolation (dysphasia)
- Depression and anxiety
- Carer stress

Before discharge, patients require routine assessment of their social circumstances and home environment. Many patients can be discharged home earlier if there is a community-based specialist team to continue with personal care assistance and rehabilitation.

Secondary prevention

All patients require a review of cardiovascular risk factors, particularly blood pressure, glucose and cholesterol levels. In the absence of a cardioembolic source, ischaemic stroke and TIA should be treated with low-dose aspirin and the addition of modified-release dipyridamole for the first 2 years according to current NICE guidelines. Clopidogrel is reserved for cases of aspirin allergy or severe intolerance. It should only be combined with aspirin when there is a cardiac indication or for a limited period under specialist supervision because of a high short-term risk of stroke after TIA.

The stroke risk following TIA can be effectively estimated by use of the ABCD^2 score (Table 4.5). Patients scoring ≥4 have a stroke risk >4% in the next 48 h and so require an urgent specialist review.

Patients with atrial fibrillation or another cardioembolic cause should be anticoagulated 2 weeks after the event unless major con-

Table 4.5 Risk of stroke after TIA (ABCD^2 score from Johnston *et al.*)

Age > 59 years	1 point
Blood pressure > 139/89 mmHg	1 point
Clinical features:	
Unilateral weakness	2 points
Speech disturbance only	1 point
Duration:	
>59 min	2 points
10–59 min	1 point
Diabetes (known)	1 point
Total	
	2 day stroke risk
High risk score (6–7)	8.1%
Moderate risk score (4–5)	4.1%
Low risk score (0–3)	1.0%

traindications are present. Screening for carotid stenosis by ultrasound should be offered to patients with carotid territory TIA and those who have recovered independence in personal care following anterior circulation ischaemic stroke (lacunar anterior circulation stroke (LACS), partial anterior circulation stroke (PACS) and total anterior circulation stroke (TACS)) within the previous 6 months.

Conclusion

Stroke and TIA are medical emergencies which require rapid assessment by a multiprofessional team. The evidence for strategies to prevent and reduce the consequences of cerebrovascular disease continues to grow, but patients and society will only benefit if specialist services are implemented and accessed in a timely manner.

Further reading

Johnston SC, Rothwell PM, Nguyen-Huynh MN *et al.* Validation and refinement of scores to predict very early stroke risk after transient ischaemic attack. *Lancet* 2007;**369**:283–292.

Nor AM, Davis J, Sen B *et al.* The Recognition of Stroke in the Emergency Room (ROSIER) scale: development and validation of a stroke recognition instrument. *Lancet Neurol* 2005;**4**:727–734.

Royal College of Physicians. *National Clinical Guidelines for Stroke*, 2nd edn. Prepared by the Intercollegiate Stroke Working Party. RCP, London, 2004.

Stroke Unit Trialists' Collaboration. Organised inpatient (stroke unit) care for stroke. *Cochrane Database Syst Rev* 2007;(4):CD000197.

Wardlaw JM, del Zoppo G, Yamaguchi T, *et al.* Thrombolysis for acute ischaemic stroke. *Cochrane Database Syst Rev* 2003;(3):CD000213.

CHAPTER 5

Carotid Artery Disease

A Ross Naylor

OVERVIEW

- Carotid endarterectomy (CEA) is of proven benefit in the management of selected patients with symptomatic and asymptomatic carotid artery disease.

- Carotid angioplasty with stenting (CAS) is an emerging alternative to CEA. The 2007 Cochrane Review does not, however, support any change from the existing recommendation that CEA remains the preferred therapeutic option outwith randomized trials.

- 'Best medical therapy' must be administered to all patients undergoing CEA or CAS.

- Delay to surgery after onset of symptoms greatly lessens the benefit conferred by CEA. If the delay exceeds 12 weeks, virtually no benefit accrues to the patient.

- The UK Department of Health has recently recommended that hospitals should consider revising practices so that CEA can be undertaken in stable, symptomatic patients within <48 h of onset of symptoms.

Introduction

In 2002, ~291 million general practitioner (GP) consultations took place in the UK. However, a General Practice Partnership caring for ~6000 patients will only see about three patients suffering a TIA and 12 with a stroke during any calendar year. Clearly, this represents an extremely small number of patients to be identified (per GP) amidst a myriad of other deserving presentations and conditions.

Previously, stroke was low in terms of public, political and professional prominence (compared with cancer and heart disease). This attitude is now changing, partly because of a new political impetus, but also because there is increasing evidence that the rapid institution of medical and surgical treatment in TIA/stroke patients really can make a difference.

In the future, the family doctor will have a key role in the management of these patients, specifically with regard to the rapid

ABC of Arterial & Venous Disease, 2nd edn. Edited by R. Donnelly and N. London. © 2009 Blackwell Publishing Ltd. 9781405178891.

referral of patients. The previous chapter focused on the medical management of cerebral vascular disease. This chapter will highlight the evidence supporting the roles of interventions such as carotid endarterectomy (CEA) and carotid angioplasty with stenting (CAS).

Aetiology of stroke/TIA

Approximately 50% of ischaemic, carotid territory TIAs or strokes follow thromboembolism of atherothrombotic debris from a stenosing plaque in the extracranial internal carotid artery (Figures 5.1 and 5.2). The first major branch of the internal carotid artery is the ophthalmic artery. Embolization into the ophthalmic artery may cause amaurosis fugax, which is usually described as a temporary 'curtain coming up or down'. Alternatively, the patient may present with a permanent altitudinal visual defect or monocular blindess (Figure 5.3). The major continuation of the internal carotid artery is the middle cerebral artery (MCA); less frequently embolic material from the internal carotid artery (ICA) may enter the anterior cerebral artery. Embolization from the ICA most commonly leads therefore to a temporary (defined as a TIA if <24 h) or permanent focal neurological defect in the MCA territory (Table 5.1). Less commonly, the anterior cerebral artery or both anterior and middle cerebral arteries are affected.

CEA removes the plaque from the ICA, while CAS involves dilatation of the stenosis with placement of a stent across the lesion. While it is important to identify patients with carotid disease (for targeting CEA and CAS), it is also important to recognize that there are other causes of ischaemic carotid territory TIAs or strokes, including small vessel intracranial disease (25%), cardiac embolism (15%), haematological (5%) and miscellaneous causes (5%).

Who benefits from CEA or CAS?

Any patient who presents with 'classical' carotid territory symptoms might benefit from carotid intervention. Most importantly, the decision to refer patients into hospital should not be based on age or the presence/absence of a carotid bruit, and no patient should simply be 'treated with aspirin' and only referred into hospital if a second event happens.

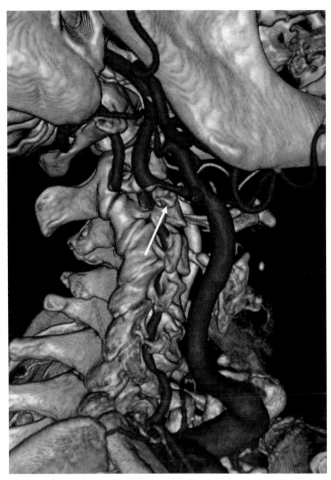

Figure 5.1 Three-dimensional CT angiogram showing a severe stenosis of the internal carotid artery (arrowed) just distal to the bifurcation

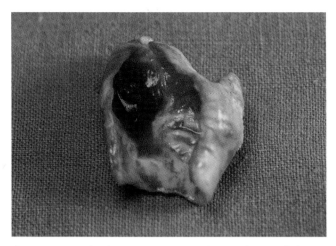

Figure 5.2 Carotid endarterectomy specimen showing the excised plaque with overlying thrombus. Embolization of this thrombotic material is responsible for 50% of ischaemic carotid territory TIAs and strokes

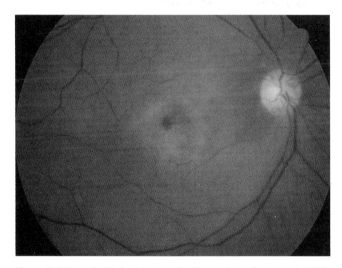

Figure 5.3 Central retinal artery occlusion in a patient who presented with sudden monocular blindness. The retina is pale with attenuated vessels. Only the fovea is spared, which appears as a cherry red spot

Table 5.1 Carotid artery TIA or stroke symptoms

Arterial territory	Area supplied	Resulting syndrome
Opthalmic artery	Retina	Amaurosis fugax, monocular altitudinal visual defect, monocular blindness
Middle cerebral artery	Parietal lobe, frontal lobe, superior temporal lobe	Contralateral facial paresis/anaesthesia, hemiplegia/hemianaesthesia (arm > leg), hemianopia, dysphasia (if dominant hemisphere), sensory inattention, visual inattention or neglect
Anterior cerebral artery frontal lobe	Anterior and superior medial	Contralateral foot and leg hemiplegia/hemianaesthesia (leg > arm)

Symptoms not due to carotid artery TIA or stroke
- Loss of or reduced consciousness
- Bilateral concurrent blurring/misting of vision
- Fainting
- Dizzyness
- Vertigo
- Amnesia.

Table 5.2 Summary of recommendations for 'best medical therapy' in patients with symptomatic carotid disease derived from the European Stroke Initiative

Treatment	Evidence grade
BP <140/90 mmHg or <130/80 mmHg in diabetic	Level I
Glycaemic control to prevent other diabetic complications	Llevel III
Statin therapy	Level I
Stop smoking	Level II
Avoid heavy consumption of alcohol	Level I
Regular physical activity	Level II
Low-salt, low-saturated fat, high-fruit and vegetable diet rich in fibre	Level II
If BMI elevated, reduce weight	Level II
HRT should not be used for stroke prevention in women	Level I
Aspirin	Level I
Aspirin and dipyridamole	Level I
Clopidogrel	Level I

Level I = evidence obtained from at least one properly designed randomized controlled trial; level II = evidence obtained from well-designed controlled trials without randomization, cohort or case–control analytic studies; level III = opinions of respected authorities, based on clinical experience.
BMI = body mass index; HRT = hormone replacement therapy.

Most hospitals now provide dedicated cerebrovascular clinics (preferably with 'single visit' imaging) and it is anticipated that these initiatives will improve to embrace 'Walk-in Clinics' in order to meet the Government's latest ambitions for speeding up the investigation and management process for stroke and TIA patients. 'Walk-in Clinics' will not, however, work if they simply become a 'funny turn' service.

When should best medical therapy start?

Irrespective of whether your patient might benefit from CEA or CAS, all should be commenced on 'best medical therapy'. Medical management has changed dramatically over the last 10 years, and Table 5.2 summarizes the current advice (and levels of evidence) from the 2004 European Stroke Initiative. More recently, the EXPRESS Study has shown that *very rapid* commencement of statin and antiplatelet therapy significantly reduces the risk of recurrent stroke, suggesting that once a diagnosis of TIA/minor stroke is made by the GP these therapies should be commenced at the time of referral to the cerebrovascular clinic.

What is the evidence for treating symptomatic patients with CEA or CAS?

CEA is one of the most scientifically scrutinized procedures of all time. Table 5.3 summarizes the principle outcomes from the Carotid Endarterectomy Trialists Collaboration (CETC) who combined data from >6000 patients randomized into the three main symptomatic trials. Table 5.3 also includes parallel data from the two multicentre randomized trials (ACAS and ACST) comparing outcomes in asymptomatic patients.

The main messages are as follows. While the symptomatic and asymptomatic trials provided level 1 evidence supporting the role of CEA in selected patients, it has to be recognized that the operation is associated with a small but important risk of peri-operative stroke/death. The key to optimizing the long-term benefit from surgery is ensuring that the initial risk is kept to the absolute minimum.

Symptomatic patients

In symptomatic patients, the CETC observed that CEA conferred a modest but significant benefit in patients with 50–69% stenoses.

Table 5.3 Carotid Endarterectomy Trialists Collaboration: 5-year risk of stroke (including 30-day stroke/death) from (i) the CETC analysis of the symptomatic randomized trials and (ii) the ACAS and ACST asymptomatic randomized trials

Trial	Stenosis	30-day CEA risk	5-year risk Surgery	Medical	RRR	NNT	Strokes prevented per 1000 CEAs
CETC	<30%		18.4%	15.7%	n/b	n/b	None at 5 years
CETC	30–49%	6.7%	22.8%	25.4%	10%	38	26 at 5 years
CETC	50–69%	8.4%	20.0%	27.8%	28%	13	78 at 5 years
CETC	70–99%	6.2%	17.1%	32.7%	48%	6	156 at 5 years
CETC	String sign	5.4%	22.4%	22.3%	n/b	n/b	None at 5 years
ACST	60–99%	2.8%	6.4%	11.8%	46%	19	53 at 5 years
ACAS	60–99%	2.3%	5.1%	11.0%	54%	17	59 at 5 years

30-day CEA risk = 30-day risk of death/stroke after CEA; n/b = no benefit conferred by CEA; RRR = relative risk reduction; NNT = number needed to treat to prevent one stroke; strokes prevented per 1000 CEAs = number of strokes prevented at 5 years by performing 1000 CEAs.

Table 5.4 CETC: effect of delay from randomization to surgery on actual benefit conferred by CEA

	<2 weeks	2–4 weeks	4–12 weeks	>12 weeks
ARR at 5 years	18.5%	9.8%	5.5%	0.8%
NNT at 5 years	5	10	18	125

ARR at 5 years = absolute risk reduction in stroke conferred by CEA at 5 years compared with best medical therapy; NNT = number of CEAs to be performed to prevent one stroke at 5 years.

This equates to relative risk reduction (RRR) =28%, number needed to treat (NNT) = 13, and 78 strokes will be prevented at 5 years by performing 1000 CEAs. The maximum benefit, however, was observed in patients with 70–99% stenoses (RRR = 48%, NNT = 6, and 156 strokes will be prevented at 5 years by performing 1000 CEAs).

One of the most important subgroup analyses to come from the CETC (Table 5.4) was recognition that while the trials recruited patients who had been symptomatic within the preceding 6 months, the maximum benefit (overall) was observed in patients who had undergone surgery within 2 weeks of randomization. The absolute relative risk (ARR) in stroke at 5 years was 18.5% in patients undergoing surgery within 2 weeks (NNT = 5), falling to just 0.8% if surgery was deferred for >12 weeks (NNT = 125). Moreover, females gained much less benefit (than males) from CEA, especially if surgery was deferred for >4 weeks. Table 5.5 summarizes other secondary analyses from the international randomized trials that identified patients who gained most benefit from intervention.

Table 5.5 Which symptomatic patients gain most benefit from carotid endarterectomy?

Clinical features	Imaging features
Males vs females	Ulcerated/irregular stenoses
Hemispheric vs retinal symptoms	Increasing stenosis (but not near occlusion)
Recurrent symptoms for >6 months	Contralateral occlusion
Very recent symptoms (2 weeks)	Tandem intracranial disease
Increasing medical co-morbidity	
Increasing age	
Very rapid surgery	

The main 'take home' messages in symptomatic patients are: (1) the prognosis of patients exhibiting near occlusion (string sign) was not as bad as had been previously anticipated. These patients do not seem to benefit from CEA. (2) The quicker the operation is performed, the greater the long-term benefit. Excessive delays will expose some patients to all of the procedural risks with little prospect of benefit. (3) Age is no bar to surgery. In the international trials, patients aged >75 years gained more benefit than any other age group. (4) The two main predictors of benefit from CEA (other than rapid surgery) were the presence of contralateral occlusion and plaque irregularity. Finally, the higher the 30-day risk, the less the long-term benefit. All surgical units must therefore maintain a rigorous audit of outcomes. The 30-day death/stroke rates

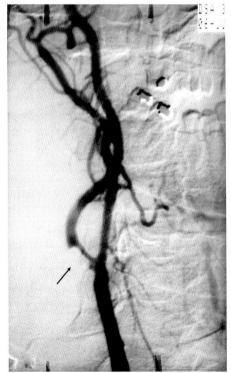 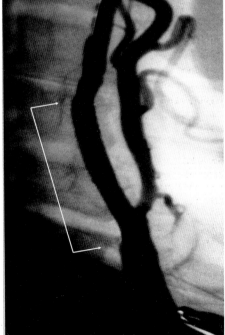

(a) (b)

Figure 5.4 (a) Pre-angioplasty angiogram showing severe internal carotid artery stenosis (arrowed) treated by percutaneous angioplasty and stenting (b, arrowed)

Table 5.6 Summary of principle findings from the 2007 Cochrane Review evaluating 12 randomized trials comparing CEA with CAS

	OR	95% CI	P-value	Heterogeneity	Comments
30-day outcomes					
Death/any stroke	1.39	1.05–1.84	0.02	No	Significantly favours CEA
Death/disabling stroke	1.22	0.83–1.79	0.31	No	No significant difference
Death	0.99	0.5–1.97	0.98	No	No significant difference
Stroke	1.40	1.02–1.91	0.04	Yes	Significantly favours CEA
Cranial nerve injury	0.07	0.03–0.20	<0.00001	No	Significantly favours CAS
Death/stroke/myocardial infarction	1.11	0.77–1.60	0.57	Yes	No significant difference
Late outcomes					
Death/stroke (including peri-operative)	1.13	0.81–1.58	0.47	Yes	No significant difference

An odds ratio (OR) of <1.0 'favours' CAS, while an OR >1.0 'favours' CEA. However, for an end-point to be statistically significant, both 95% confidence intervals (CIs) must be either <1.0 (i.e. CAS is significantly better) or >1.0 (i.e. CEA is significantly better). There was marked heterogeneity between some of the studies due to different types of patients, CAS techniques and length of follow-up.

should be <5% in standard risk symptomatic patients and <3% in asymptomatic individuals.

Asymptomatic patients

In asymptomatic patients, both ACAS and ACST showed that immediate CEA (as opposed to deferred CEA) was associated with a small but significant reduction in the risk of late stroke, from ~12% at 5 years to ~6% (Table 5.3). On average, 18 patients need to undergo surgery to prevent one stroke at 5 years and, provided the 30-day risk remains <2.5%, approximately 56 strokes will be prevented at 5 years by performing 1000 operations.

Clearly, the benefit from CEA is much less in asymptomatic patients. Few secondary analyses have been performed on the ACAS and ACST cohorts. The available 'take home' messages are: (1) CEA does not appear to confer benefit in patients aged >75 years. (2) Women do not gain as much benefit as men. The significant benefit reported in ACST was only present in women if the 30-day death/stroke risk was excluded. It does seem likely, however, that when the 10-year data are released, there will be evidence of benefit in the younger female, perhaps aged <70 years. (3) There is no apparent association between late stroke risk and either ipsilateral stenosis severity or contralateral occlusion.

CEA or CAS?

CAS (Figure 5.4) has emerged as a non-invasive alternative to CEA, and quoted advantages include no neck incision, no cranial nerve injuries, shorter hospital stay and improved cost-effectiveness. It is inevitable that CAS and CEA will have a complementary role but, to date, a number of randomized trials have failed to establish consensus.

Table 5.6 summarizes the principle findings from the 2007 Cochrane Review which now includes 12 randomized trials (3227 patients). As can be seen, several 30-day outcomes were significantly in favour of CEA (death/stroke, stroke), while the lack of cranial nerve injury was heavily in favour of CAS. A number of end-points showed no statistical significance (death/disabling stroke, death, death/stroke/myocardial infarction). Long term, the data are difficult to interpret, but there does not seem to be a significant difference in late stroke risk.

The authors of this Cochrane Review concluded that the current data do not support a move away from recommending CEA as the first-line treatment of choice without participation in randomized trials. This review will be soon be updated when two very large (and nearly completed) randomized trials report. It is expected that the addition of almost 4000 patients will greatly inform the debate.

Further reading

Ederle J, Featherstone RL, Brown MM. Percutaneous transluminal angioplasty and stenting for carotid artery stenosis. *Cochrane Database Syst Rev* 2007;4:CD000515.

European Stroke Initiative Executive Committee; EUSI Writing Committee. European Stroke Initiative Recommendations for stroke management—Update 2003. *Cerebrovasc Dis* 2003;16:311–337.

Naylor AR. Time is brain! *The Surgeon* 2007;5:23–30.

Rothwell PM, Eliasziw M, Gutnikov SA *et al.* for the Carotid Endarterectomy Trialists Collaboration. Endarterectomy for symptomatic carotid stenosis in relation to clinical subgroups and timing of surgery. *Lancet* 2004:363:915–924.

Rothwell PM, Giles MF, Chandratheva A *et al.* Effect of urgent treatment of transient ischaemic attack and minor stroke on early recurrent stroke (EXPRESS study): a prospective population-based sequential comparison. *Lancet* 2007;370:1432–1442.

CHAPTER 6

Diabetes and Vascular Disease

Garry Tan, Richard Donnelly

OVERVIEW

- There is a significant impact of diabetes on health: 2.4% of all deaths can be attributed to diabetes and 5% of all NHS expenditure (9% of all hospital costs).

- Diabetic vascular diseases can be divided into two categories: microvascular complications and macrovascular complications.

- The functional and structural changes associated with microangiopathy include thickening of the capillary basement membrane, increased permeability to macromolecules (e.g. causing proteinuria and macular oedema) and microvascular ischaemia due to thrombotic occlusion.

- In the United Kingdom Prospective Diabetes Study (UKPDS)—a landmark trial in patients with type 2 diabetes mellitus—intensive glucose control reduces the risk of microvascular complications in type 1 and type 2 diabetes by 25–30%.

- Diabetic retinopathy is the most common cause of blindness in people aged 30–69 years.

- A patient with diabetes and proteinuria has a mortality rate which is 40 times higher than that of a diabetic patient without proteinuria.

- In diabetes, the risk of ischaemic stroke is increased by 2- to 4-fold, although the rate of haemorrhagic strokes is similar to that of the general population.

Diabetes affects 4.67% of people in the UK and its prevalence is increasing (5.05% by 2010). There is a significant impact on health: 2.4% of all deaths can be attributed to diabetes and 5% of all NHS expenditure (9% of all hospital costs).

The life expectancy of someone with diabetes is reduced by an average of 5–10 years, with an annual mortality rate of 5.4% (double the rate of people without diabetes). Vascular diseases are the principal causes of death and disability in people with diabetes (Table 6.1).

ABC of Arterial & Venous Disease, 2nd edn. Edited by R. Donnelly and N. London.
© 2009 Blackwell Publishing Ltd. 9781405178891.

Diabetic vascular diseases can be divided into two categories: microvascular complications and macrovascular complications (Table 6.2).

Microvascular disease

Diabetes can affect the smallest blood vessels in the body (the capillary and pre-capillary arterioles). The functional and structural changes associated with microangiopathy include thickening of the capillary basement membrane, increased permeability to macromolecules (e.g. causing proteinuria and macular oedema) and microvascular ischaemia due to thrombotic occlusion. These changes result in damage to the eyes, kidneys, peripheral nerves and even the heart.

Blood sugars and microvascular disease

The development and progression of microvascular complications are intimately linked to elevated blood sugar levels. In fact, the diagnosis of diabetes is partly based on the level of blood glucose concentrations at which microvascular complications (such as diabetic retinopathy) develop.

Lowering blood sugar levels reduces the risk of microvascular complications in patients with type 1 (T1DM) and type 2 diabetes mellitus (T2DM). For every 1% reduction in glycated haemoglobin (HbA$_{1c}$), there is ~25–35% reduction in microvascular disease. For example, in the Diabetes Control and Complications Trial (DCCT)—a landmark study in T1DM—intensive insulin treatment over 9 years was associated with a reduction in the number of microvascular complications by 34–76%. The intensively treated group reduced their HbA$_{1c}$ from 8 to 7.2%, and long-term follow-up of these patients (long after the randomized part of the study finished) has shown a lasting benefit from intensive glycaemic control in the early years after diagnosis.

In the United Kingdom Prospective Diabetes Study (UKPDS)—a landmark trial in patients with T2DM—intensive glucose control over 10 years was associated with a reduction in the number of microvascular complications by 25%. The tight glucose control group reduced their HbA$_{1c}$ by an average of 0.9% more than the comparator group. However, lower blood sugars and lower HbA$_{1c}$s have been associated with an increased risk of severe

Table 6.1 Risk of morbidity associated with diabetes (all types)

Complication	Relative risk compared with people without diabetes
Blindness	20
End-stage renal disease	25
Amputation	40
Peripheral vascular disease	4
Myocardial infarction	2–5
Stroke	2–3

Table 6.2 Vascular complications of diabetes

Microvascular	Macrovascular
Retinopathy	Ischaemic heart disease
Nephropathy	Stroke
Neuropathy	Peripheral vascular disease

hypoglycaemia (i.e. hypoglycaemia needing help from a third party), and this must be balanced against the benefits of tight glycaemic control in individual patients.

Diabetic retinopathy

Diabetic retinopathy is the most common cause of blindness in people aged 30–69 years. Twenty years after diagnosis, nearly all people with T1DM, and 80% of those with T2DM, will have some degree of diabetic retinopathy.

Diabetes causes a range of ophthalmological complications including corneal abnormalities, glaucoma, iris neovascularization and cataracts. Initially, patients are generally asymptomatic, although symptoms such as blurred vision, visual distortion or visual acuity loss can occur in more advanced disease.

Diabetic retinopathy can be examined using an ophthalmoscope (a red-free filter, i.e. a green filter, helps to make haemorrhages and new vessels easier to see), a slit lamp or digital photography. In the UK, national screening programmes are being implemented to offer regular retinopathy screening to every adult with diabetes (Table 6.3).

Microaneurysms are the first sign of diabetic retinopathy. These are aneurysmal swellings of capillary walls and appear as small red dots. *Small blot haemorrhages* are produced as microaneurysms rupture, whilst *flame-shaped haemorrhages* represent bleeding in more superficial nerve fibre layers. As the blood–retinal barrier breaks down, leakage of proteins and lipids produce *hard exudates* which can themselves be threatening to vision if they occur in the region of the macula (an exudative *maculopathy*). The macula can also become ischaemic if there is a predominance of capillary occlusion (an ischaemic maculopathy). Extensive leakage at the macula can lead to macula oedema (an oedematous maculopathy).

Hard exudates appear as waxy or yellowish white deposits and are seen as individual spots, clusters or streaks, or as large 'circinate' rings around collections of microaneurysms or damaged capillaries. Other changes of diabetes include *cotton wool spots* (due to nerve fibre infarction and formerly known as soft exudates) and

venous abnormalities (venous loops, duplication or beading which precede the development of new vessel formation). *Intraretinal microvascular abnormalities* (IRMAs—on the borders of ischaemic retina) are tortuous abnormally shaped capillaries which are present within areas of retinal ischaemia and signify pre-proliferative retinopathy.

Vision-threatening retinopathy is usually due to new vessel formation in T1DM and to maculopathy in T2DM. Patients with active proliferative diabetic retinopathy should not be given thrombolytic drugs because they are at increased risk of retinal haemorrhage. There is no evidence of increased risk of retinal bleeding with aspirin therapy.

Treatment of diabetic eye disease involves laser treatment or vitrectomy. Diabetic maculopathy and proliferative retinopathy are treated with laser photocoagulation to prevent further loss of vision rather than to restore diminished acuity. Vitrectomy may improve vision after a vitreous haemorrhage, retinal detachment or scarring. Prevention of diabetic eye disease is based around regular checks and good blood pressure and blood glucose control. New treatments such as intravitreal injections of vascular endothelial growth factor (VEGF) inhibitors are under assessment, and there is some evidence that lipid-lowering therapy using statins may also have a beneficial effect on retinopathy progression.

Nephropathy

Diabetic nephropathy is the commonest cause of end-stage renal disease (ESRD) in Western countries, accounting for >25% of people entering renal replacement therapy. It is also associated with significant morbidity and mortality: a patient with diabetes and proteinuria has a mortality rate which is 40 times higher than that of a diabetic patient without proteinuria.

There are some differences between the nephropathies which occur in T1DM and in T2DM:

- microalbuminuria is less predictive of progression of nephropathy in T2DM than in T1DM patients
- hypertension is more common in T2DM nephropathy
- in T2DM, albuminuria is more likely to be present at diagnosis of diabetes.

Diabetic nephropathy usually develops after diabetes has been present for at least 10 years. Risk factors for nephropathy include male sex, age, smoking status and glycaemic control. The peak incidence (3% per annum) occurs after diabetes has been present for 10–20 years; the incidence declines thereafter.

Initially, diabetic nephropathy is associated with an increased glomerular filtration rate (GFR). As nephropathy progresses, the GFR decreases and microalbuminuria (30–300 mg of albumin/day) develops. Macroalbuminuria (>300 mg of albumin/day) and hypertension then follow as the GFR falls below the normal range. Without specific interventions, ~80% of people with T1DM and 20–40% of people with T2DM with microalbuminuria will progress to overt albuminuria. Because early treatment can prevent the progression of diabetic nephropathy, screening for early nephropathy with urinalysis is recommended. In a random urine sample, the microalbumin:creatinine ratio can be measured. A ratio of <2.5 (albumin in µg/creatinine in mmol) is normal in women and <3.5 is normal in men. At least two measurements should be made

Table 6.3 Classification of diabetic retinopathy by the English National Screening Programme

Grade	Description	Symptoms	Observed change
Retinopathy			
R0	No retinopathy	None	None
R1	Background (or mild/moderate non-proliferative) retinopathy	None	Microaneurysm(s)
			Retinal haemorrhage(s) ± hard exudate(s)
R2	Pre-proliferative (or severe non-proliferative) retinopathy	None	Venous beading
			Venous loop(s) or reduplication
			Intraretinal microvascular abnormality (IRMA)
			Multiple deep, round or blot haemorrhages
			Cotton wool spots
R3	Proliferative	Floaters, sudden visual loss, central loss of vision	New vessels at the disc
			New vessels elsewhere (NVE)
			Pre-retinal, vitreous haemorrhages
			Pre-retinal fibrosis ± tractional retinal detachment
Maculopathy			
M0	No maculopathy	None	
M1	Maculopathy	Blurred central vision	Exudate within 1 disc diameter (DD) of the centre of the fovea
			Circinate or group of exudates within the macula
			Any microaneurysm or haemorrhage within 1 DD of the centre of the fovea if associated with a
			best visual acuity of ≤6/12
			Ischaemic maculopathy can produce featureless macula with NVE and poor vision
Photocoagulation			
P0	No photocoagulation		
P1	Photocoagulation	Reduced night vision, glare	Focal/grid laser therapy to macula
			Peripheral scatter laser therapy
Unclassifiable			
U			Often because of cataracts obscuring view of retina

Note: a patient will be given a grade in each of the three categories. For example, a patient might be classified as R2 M1 P0. Other UK national screening grading systems have different grades.

before microalbuminuria is diagnosed. Microalbuminuria itself is an independent predictor of cardiovascular morbidity and mortality.

Renal biopsies are not routinely indicated in all cases of diabetic nephropathy. If the history and progression are atypical then a biopsy might be indicated, e.g. if the duration of diabetes is short, if there is no proteinuria or if other associated manifestations of diabetes, such as retinopathy, are absent.

Hyperglycaemia is closely linked with the progression of diabetic nephropathy, and tight glycaemic control may slow progression even after overt proteinuria has developed. Tight blood pressure control also slows diabetic nephropathy progression. Angiotensin-converting enzyme (ACE) inhibitors or angiotensin II receptor blockers (ARBs) probably confer benefits over and above blood pressure reduction, and ARBs have evidence of renoprotection especially in T2DM nephropathy. The combination treatment of ACE inhibitors and ARBs does not appear to offer greater renoprotection and may in fact accelerate disease progression.

If ESRD develops, haemodialysis, peritoneal dialysis, renal transplantation or combined kidney–pancreas transplantation are treatment options. Patients with diabetic nephropathy tend to develop anaemia at higher GFRs than people with other causes of renal disease. This may relate to decreased erythropoietin production with an autonomic neuropathy (which is common in diabetes).

Care must be taken with radiographic dyes as their use can precipitate acute renal failure in patients with underlying diabetic nephropathy. Metformin should be discontinued in patients before such studies, and N-acetylcysteine may be used for renoprotection prior to contrast administration. Metformin should be avoided in patients with a creatinine >150 µmol/l because of the increased risk of lactic acidosis.

Box 6.1 **Classification of diabetic neuropathies**

Hyperglycaemic neuropathies
Generalized neuropathies
- Sensorimototr polyneuropathy
- Acute painful sensory neuropathy
- Autonomic neuropathy
- Acute motor neuropathy

Focal and multifocal neuropathies
- Cranial neuropathies
- Thoracolumbar radiculopathy
- Proximal diabetic neuropathy

Focal limb neuropathies (includes entrapment and compression neuropathies)

Table 6.4 Clinical features that distinguish neuropathic and vascular foot ulcers

Neuropathic	Vascular
Painless	Painful
Located at points of high pressure	Often located at extremities
'Punched out' appearance surrounded by callus	
Warm foot	Cool ischaemic foot
Bounding foot pulses	Absent foot pulses

Neuropathies

Neuropathies are the most common complication of diabetes (with a prevalence of up to 50%) (Box 6.1). They cause significant morbidity when painful and also lead to secondary problems such as falls, foot ulcers and cardiac arrhythmias.

A symmetrical sensorimotor neuropathy is most common (usually with a predominant sensory component). It occurs in a glove-and-stocking distribution. Besides causing significant pain, this type of neuropathy eventually results in the loss of peripheral sensation. The combination of decreased sensation and peripheral arterial insufficiency often leads to foot ulceration and eventually amputation of toes or part of the lower limb. Feet at high risk of ulceration should be identified for specialist advice and intervention (Box 6.2).

The pain of diabetic neuropathy can be treated with many drugs including amitriptyline, sodium valproate, gabapentin/pregabalin and topical capsaicin. In general, an asymmetrical distribution, predominant motor component and greater involvement of the hands than the feet are features that should prompt further investigation for other causes. The features of neuropathic ulcers are summarized in Table 6.4.

Of the cranial neuropathies, the third cranial nerve is most commonly affected (the pupil is spared, the ptosis is partial and there is no pain in a diabetic (medical) third nerve palsy; whereas in a surgical third nerve palsy the pupil is dilated, the ptosis total and is painful, such as that caused by an intracranial aneurysm). They usually resolve spontaneously in several months. However, >40%

Box 6.2 **Clinical features of the 'high risk' diabetic foot**

- Impaired sensation (monofilament)
- Past or current ulcer
- Maceration
- Fungal or gryphotic (thickened or horny) toenails
- Biomechanical problems (corns or callus)
- Fissures
- Clawed toes

of third nerve palsies in people with diabetes are due to causes other than diabetes and should therefore be investigated.

Autonomic dysfunction can involve any sympathetic or parasympathetic function. Common symptoms include nausea and vomiting (due to gastroparesis—look for other causes, rehydrate and treat with small regular meals, metoclopramide and erythromycin, parenteral nutrition or even gastric pacing) and postural hypotension (treat with simple advice on standing up slowly, support stockings or fludrocortisone).

Macrovascular disease

Atheroma in patients with diabetes is identical at a microscopic level to that found in people without diabetes. However, atherosclerosis tends to be more diffusely distributed and its course over time differs: it tends to begin at an earlier age and to progress more rapidly than in people without diabetes. Plaque rupture is more common. The reasons for these differences are unclear and have been attributed to abnormalities in platelets, vascular function, clotting, red cell function, lipids and protein, perhaps highlighting the fact that diabetes is an abnormality of metabolism, of which abnormal glucose control is only one facet.

Treating risk factors for cardiovascular disease

To delay the progression of diabetic cardiovascular disease (CVD), co-existent risk factors should be aggressively identified and treated. Smoking status, blood glucose control, blood pressure and plasma lipid concentrations should be assessed at least annually.

Secondary prevention and the treatment of risk factors

In people with diabetes who are known to have CVD, the importance of lipid-lowering therapy is well established. A 1 mmol/l reduction in total or low-density lipoprotein (LDL)-cholesterol reduces CVD risk by 36%. People with diabetes and known CVD are at a much higher risk (>2-fold) of further events compared with people with CVD but no diabetes, emphasizing the importance of aggressive management. The use of aspirin in secondary prevention in patients with diabetes is generally supported by the literature, although it is unclear as to the optimum dose (*in vitro* studies of aspirin on platelet thromboxane levels suggest that higher doses might be needed—something not studied clinically). In acute coronary syndromes, aspirin is combined with clopidogrel.

Primary prevention and the treatment of risk factors

Aspirin's role in the *primary* prevention of CVD is controversial. Many guidelines recommend its use in people over the age of 40 with well controlled hypertension. However, this is supported by few data, and large ongoing multicentre trials are addressing this issue in both T1DM and T2DM.

It has been usual to manage everyone with T2DM as if for secondary rather than primary prevention of CVD. Practically, this has meant the widespread prescribing of statin therapy in everyone with T2DM over the age of 40, irrespective of their starting lipid levels. Statin use in patients under the age of 40 is still recommended for those at highest CVD risk. Of course, particular care must be taken in the use of statins in women of childbearing potential.

Most guidelines do not differentiate between T1DM and T2DM in their use of lipid-lowering therapies in primary prevention of CVD. However, it should be noted that people with T1DM do not share the same lipid profile as those with T2DM (which is associated with low concentrations of high-density lipoprotein (HDL)-cholesterol and high concentrations of small dense atherogenic LDL-cholesterol).

Glycaemic control and macrovascular disease

A 1% reduction in HbA_{1c} is associated with a reduction in the risk of myocardial infarction by 14%. However, at the time of writing, there is controversy over whether or not there is an increase in mortality in T2DM patients with pre-existing CVD or with multiple CVD risk factors when they are targeted for very intensive lowering of HbA_{1c} to <6.5%. Results from three large studies investigating the benefits and risks of very tight glycaemic control in T2DM are soon to be published (the ACCORD, ADVANCE and ORIGIN studies).

Cerebrovascular disease

In the general population, ~85% of strokes are ischaemic and 15% are haemorrhagic (10% primary intracerebral haemorrhage and 5% subarachnoid haemorrhage). In diabetes, the risk of ischaemic stroke is increased by 2- to 4-fold, although the rate of haemorrhagic strokes is similar to that of the general population (Figure 6.1). Following a stroke, a patient with diabetes is more likely to die or suffer severe residual disability. Glucose control is important in

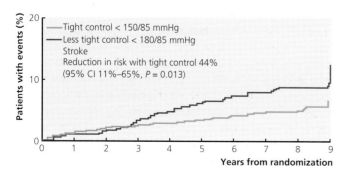

Figure 6.1 Kaplan–Meier plot of the proportion of patients who developed fatal or non-fatal stroke according to blood pressure. Adapted from UK Prospective Diabetes Study Group (1998)

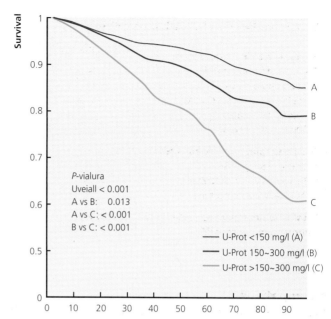

Figure 6.2 Proteinuria predicts stroke survival. In addition, this study reported stroke incidence as 7.2% in diabetic patients without proteinuria, 11.1% in those with borderline proteinuria and 23.0% in those with clinical proteinuria (versus the corresponding rates among non-diabetic subjects of 1.6%, 3.2% and 8.5%, respectively. Adapted from Miettinen *et al.* (1996)

the acute phases of stroke, and otherwise treatment should be the same as for patients without diabetes (Figure 6.2). Diabetes is also a risk factor for vascular dementia, increasing the risk by 2- to 3-fold. Treatment (and prevention) is the same as that for non-diabetic patients.

Ischaemic heart disease

CVD accounts for 75% of deaths in T2DM and 35% in T1DM. Patients with diabetes may present with classical symptoms of cardiac ischaemia, but often the presentation includes atypical symptoms such as sweating, malaise, dyspnoea or syncope (often confused with hypoglycaemia). Silent ischaemia is more common in diabetes and has a worse prognosis. Diastolic dysfunction is also common in patients with diabetes and should be considered in the patient with symptoms of congestive heart failure and a normal ejection fraction.

Use of β-blockers after a myocardial infarction in a patient with diabetes reduces mortality, sudden death and non-fatal reinfarction. They do not increase the frequency or severity of hypoglycaemic attacks and should not be withheld from patients with diabetes (unless there is critical limb ischaemia).

Peripheral arterial disease

The presentation and treatment of peripheral arterial disease (PAD) in patients with diabetes is similar to that in people without diabetes. However, ABPIs may be falsely elevated in diabetics, and PAD tends to be more diffuse, distal and complicated in the diabetic. Angioplasty or stenting is useful for short segment occlusions (<10 cm in length) in proximal regions.

Further reading

Gries FA, Cameron NE, Low PA. *Textbook of Diabetic Neuropathy*. Thieme, Stuttgart, 2003.

Miettinen H, Haffner SM, Lehto S *et al*. Proteinuria predicts stroke and other atherosclerotic vascular disease events in nondiabetic and non-insulin-dependent diabetic subjects. *Stroke* 1996;**27**:2033–2039.

UK Prospective Diabetes Study Group. Tight blood pressure control and risk of macrovascular and microvascular complications in type 2 diabetes (UKPDS 38). *BMJ* 1998;**317**:703–713.

Wass JAH, Shalet SM. *Oxford Textbook of Endocrinology and Diabetes*. Oxford University Press, Oxford, 2002.

www.wales.nhs.uk/sites3/page.cfm?orgid=562&pid=12776

www.nscretinopathy.org.uk

www.nsd.scot.nhs.uk/services/drs/

www.diabeticretinopathy.org.uk

CHAPTER 7

Renal Artery Stenosis

Patrick B Mark, Alan G Jardine, Giles H Roditi, Adrian J Brady

OVERVIEW

- Despite advances in imaging technology that detect structural renal artery disease, the diagnosis of functional disease remains complex, and controversy remains over whether, when and how to treat atheromatous renal artery stenosis (RAS).

- Apart from difficult-to-treat hypertension, a relatively common clinical presentation of RAS is acute renal failure, particularly in patients who receive drugs that block the renin–angiotensin system. A less common presentation is recurrent, rapid-onset ('flash') pulmonary oedema.

- It is possible to obtain high-resolution CT images of the renal vessels with additional information on calcification of lesions, but the dose of radiation is substantial and the iodine-based contrast medium carries a risk of nephrotoxicity.

- The main impact of RAS is not on the development of renal failure but on poorer outcome from vascular lesions in other territories.

- The ASTRAL (Angioplasty and Stent for Renal Artery Lesions) trial randomized patients with atherosclerotic RAS (where clinical uncertainty existed as to whether revascularization was indicated) to medical therapy or stenting. Preliminary reports suggest that there is no benefit of renal artery stenting compared with medical therapy in terms of decline of renal function, blood pressure or overall vascular events.

Introduction

Stenosis of the renal artery is a common medical condition, caused by atherosclerotic vascular disease in older patients, and fibromuscular dysplasia (FMD) in young individuals. Stenosis can cause hypertension, heart failure and progressive chronic kidney disease (CKD). However, in many patients, renal artery stenosis (RAS) is silent, accompanying disseminated atherosclerotic vascular disease in other territories. Despite advances in imaging technology that detect structural renal artery disease, the diagnosis of functional

disease remains complex, and controversy remains over whether, when and how to treat atheromatous RAS (Box 7.1).

Box 7.1 **Characteristics of renal artery stenosis**

Fibromuscular dysplasia (10%)
- Younger age group
- Female preponderance
- Hypertension
- General good response to angioplasty
- Renal impairment rare
- Involves intima, media and adventitia
- Nodular stenosis

Atherosclerotic renal artery stenosis (90%)
- Older age group
- More common in men
- Smokers
- Associated with chronic kidney disease
- Presence of widespread atherosclerotic vascular disease
- Associated with/causes hypertension—often refractory

Pathophysiology

The pathophysiology of uncomplicated unilateral and bilateral RAS provides a paradigm for the development of hypertension. Narrowing of the lumen of a renal artery beyond 75% in cross-sectional area reduces renal perfusion (Figure 7.1). This activates the renin–angiotensin system and increases circulating levels of renin, angiotensin II and aldosterone. This in turn causes hypertension, mediated by the actions of angiotensin II and aldosterone, and sometimes hypokalaemia, caused by mineralocorticoid excess. These are the features of secondary hyperaldosteronism, distinguished from primary hyperaldosteronism by the presence of high plasma sodium in the latter. In experimental models, and in some patients with unilateral RAS, these features may be reversed by revascularization. However, for the majority of patients who present late, there are secondary changes within the vasculature that lead to sustained hypertension, although electrolyte abnormalities may be reversed (Box 7.2).

ABC of Arterial & Venous Disease, 2nd edn. Edited by R. Donnelly and N. London.
© 2009 Blackwell Publishing Ltd. 9781405178891.

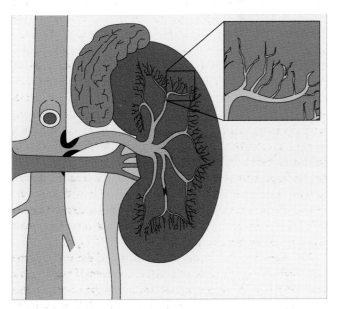

Figure 7.1 Atheromatous renal artery stenosis typically affects the origin of the main renal artery but may involve the branch, and smaller renal vessels

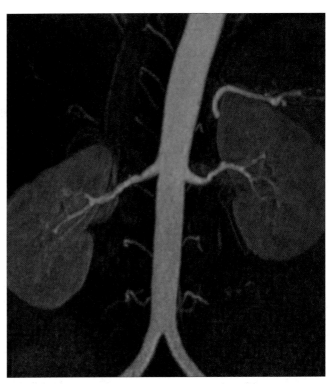

Figure 7.2 Coronal projection of contrast-enhanced MRA demonstrating renal artery stenosis due to fibromuscular dysplasia of the renal arteries. Lesions typically affect the main and branch renal arteries, are beaded in appearance and are often multifocal

In patients with bilateral RAS, levels of the components of the renin–angiotensin system are not necessarily elevated. Moreover, in treated hypertensives, antihypertensive drug therapy may mask the hormonal and electrolyte changes seen in experimental RAS, so that plasma levels of renin and aldosterone may be unhelpful or misleading. Hypertension develops as a consequence of impaired clearance of salt and water, and reduced GFR, which also causes development of heart failure, particularly in patients with bilateral disease.

Clinical features

Atheromatous RAS (ARAS) typically occurs in older patients, often male, with co-existent vascular disease in other territories and a high prevalence of conventional cardiovascular risk factors, unlike RAS due to FMD which affects younger, principally female subjects (Figure 7.2).

This is of major importance as most patients will die of vascular disease, rather than directly as a consequence of ARAS. Conventionally, RAS is associated with hypertension, typically with blood pressure that is difficult to treat; or occasionally malignant hypertension; and hypertension associated with CKD (Figure 7.3). ARAS

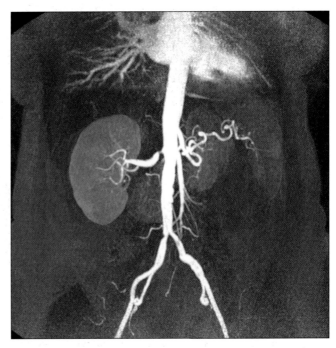

Figure 7.3 Coronal projection of contrast-enhanced MRA in a severely hypertensive patient showing a tight atherosclerotic stenosis at the origin of the right renal artery supplying a normal sized kidney. The left renal artery is also critically stenosed and the left kidney small

is also a well recognized cause of ESRD. Patients who present with renal impairment or renal failure typically have a bland urine sediment, or very low level proteinuria. Histologically, the kidneys of patients who develop ESRD due to renal artery disease show ischaemic changes, with glomerular shrinkage and tubular interstitial fibrosis, although a small number show features of focal segmental glomerular sclerosis (FSGS) which may be associated with heavy proteinuria.

Box 7.3 **Clinical features of renal artery stenosis**

- Young hypertensive patients (fibromuscular dysplasia)
- Resistant hypertension
- Widespread atherosclerosis
- Renal impairment with minimal proteinuria
- Drop in estimated glomerular filtration rate >30% with angiotensin-converting enzyme inhibition
- Pulmonary oedema despite normal left ventricular function
- >1.5 cm difference in kidney size on ultrasound
- Secondary hyperaldosteronism (low-normal plasma sodium and low potassium concentrations)

Another, relatively common clinical presentation is with acute renal failure, particularly in patients with bilateral RAS (or stenosis in a single functioning kidney) who receive drugs that block the renin–angiotensin system, precipitated by dehydration or concomitant illness. Less common presentations include recurrent, rapid-onset ('flash') pulmonary oedema, which is probably a consequence of the fluid retention and diastolic ventricular dysfunction that accompany bilateral atherosclerotic RAS.

The above features tend to be associated with large vessel RAS. However, renal impairment may occur in patients with non-critical lesions of the large vessels and diffuse disease affecting branch vessels within the renal parenchyma. Biochemical abnormalities may be present in patients in the absence of significant renal impairment. Clinical examination may reveal bruits over major vessels, including the abdominal aorta and femoral arteries that are features of widespread atherosclerosis. Lateralizing bruits in patients with unilateral renal stenosis are uncommon (Box 7.3).

Diagnosis

Atheromatous RAS should be suspected in patients with hypertension, renal impairment and atheromatous disease in other territories. The main differential diagnosis is hypertensive nephrosclerosis—uncommon in Caucasian populations—and cholesterol microembolic disease that usually follows invasive vascular procedures or anticoagulation. The differential diagnosis may be difficult, as all three can occur simultaneously. The 'gold standard' investigation for detecting structural disease is angiography, with selective renal artery cannulation, with or without digital subtraction imaging and potentially supplemented by pressure measurements across any stenosis found and/or intravascular ultrasound as angiography alone may not suffice. This requires arterial puncture, with associated risk of an invasive procedure as well as the use of nephrotoxic contrast agents. Clinical practice

has moved towards the use of non-invasive investigations, specifically computed tomographic angiography (CTA) and magnetic resonance angiography (MRA) (Figures 7.4 and 7.5). With modern multidetector row CT, it is possible to obtain high spatial resolution images of the renal vessels with additional information on calcification of lesions that may have implications for treatment. However, the dose of radiation is substantial, and the requirement for high iodine concentration contrast medium remains, with the potential for nephrotoxicity. Early non-contrast MRA techniques lacked accuracy but, with the advent of contrast-enhanced MRA (CE-MRA) with gadolinium-based contrast agents, MRA became a viable tool for renal arterial imaging. Clinical trials have shown high accuracy of CE-MRA for ostial and proximal RAS in patients with renal impairment. While contrast-enhanced MRA can depict stenotic disease in the main renal artery, the determination of its haemodynamic significance is more difficult although phase contrast MRA flow quantification has an adjunctive role for this purpose. However, the accuracy of both CTA and CE-MRA is less impressive in assessing branch RAS when compared with digital subtraction angiography (DSA) in patients with systolic hypertension. This poor accuracy for branch vessels is due to the inadequate spatial resolution of both the CT and MRI systems employed combined with vessel blurring due to motion in patients unable to breath-hold for the scan. Continued advances with both imaging modalities will address these issues, such as parallel imaging techniques and improved contrast agents with MRI, whilst submillimetre collimation fast rotation systems driven by cardiac applications have improved CTA quality.

The recent recognition of the association of the use of some gadolinium contrast agents with the development of nephrogenic systemic fibrosis in patients with severe renal impairment has also served to dampen enthusiasm for the use of CE-MRA for investigation of patients with severe renal impairment. The risks of this rare condition must be weighed against the risks of nephrotoxic iodinated contrast and ionizing radiation.

Although these tests provide structural information, they do not routinely yield information on the functional significance of RAS. CT can accurately assess enhanced renal parenchymal volume as a potential surrogate for function. MRI can give similar information, and quantitative flow techniques show great promise for the quantification of regional blood flow, though this remains in the research domain. Isotope renography, with or without the use of captopril, generates some information on the function of each kidney, but it is uncommon for this test to show clear evidence of functional RAS. Moreover, isotope renography provides little information where small vessel disease exists. Ultrasound excludes obstructive uropathy while providing information on renal size, and renal asymmetry is associated with functional disease. Simple renal size is useful information as regards the potential benefits of revascularization since kidneys <8 cm in length do not achieve useful function after revascularization. In practice, it is common to use ultrasonography as a screening test, before proceeding to either non-invasive or invasive angiography. Accurate Doppler imaging of the main renal arteries and hilar branches is technically difficult, but intrarenal vascular resistance is more easily obtained, and this measurement in the kidney not affected by RAS has

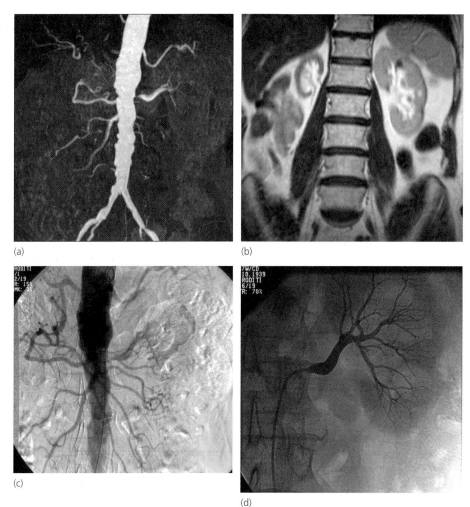

(a)   (b)

(c)   (d)

Figure 7.4 (a) Coronal projection of contrast-enhanced MRA in a patient with moderate impairment showing a tight stenosis at the origin of the left renal artery supplying a normal sized kidney. The right renal artery is occluded; the corresponding T2-weighted MRI image (b) shows the atrophic, hypointense right kidney on the side of renal artery occlusion along with preserved size and parenchymal signal of the left kidney despite the RAS. Digital subtraction angiography (c) confirms the findings at MRA, with the left renal artery stenosis assessed in more detail by selective renal artery cannulation (d)

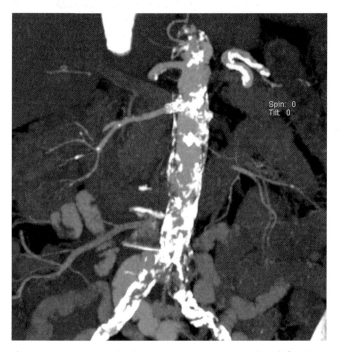

Figure 7.5 CT angiography demonstrating extensive vascular calcification. The left renal artery is occluded, with a right renal artery stent *in situ*

been shown to predict the results of revascularization. While this is of limited value as a general diagnostic test, it may be useful in the assessment and follow-up of individual cases considered for intervention (Box 7.4).

Box 7.4 **Diagnostic tests**

- Ultrasound
- MR angiography
- CT angiography
- Captopril renography
- Formal angiography

Natural history and prognosis

The natural history of ARAS, as with atheromatous stenosis in other territories, is of progressive narrowing, and ultimately occlusion. The rate of occlusion is ~5% per annum, but, like atheroma elsewhere, spontaneous plaque rupture and rapid progression may occur, with many of these patients having features of low-grade

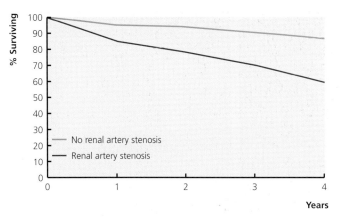

Figure 7.6 Effect of co-existent renal artery stenosis on survival among patients having coronary angiography. Data from Conlon *et al.* (1998)

cholesterol embolism heralded by the presence of peripheral eosinophilia. Patients who have bilateral RAS associated with renal artery occlusion are three times more likely to reach ESRD than patients who have bilateral disease without occlusion. Moreover, the rate of loss of renal function and progressive reduction in renal size (measured by ultrasound) is also about three times greater for patients with bilateral disease and/or occlusion.

The main impact of ARAS is not on the development of renal failure but on poorer outcome from vascular lesions in other territories. Thus, patients with coronary disease or peripheral vascular disease and ARAS have a reduced life expectancy. Whether this is a consequence of reduced renal excretory function—which is an independent predictor of premature cardiovascular death—or a marker for the severity of widespread atherosclerotic vascular disease is not clear. In fact, most of the data come from studies where the renal arteries have been imaged as the coronary artery catheter is removed following coronary artery catheterization. This procedure—commonly known as 'drive-by shooting'—reveals a high prevalence of atherosclerotic RAS in patients with coronary disease (Figure 7.6).

Box 7.5 **Medical treatment of atherosclerotic renal artery stenosis**

- Smoking cessation
- Lipid-lowering therapy
- Antiplatelet agents
- Drugs to reduce blood pressure (angiotensin-converting enzyme inhibitors only under specialist advice)

Treatment (Box 7.5)

Over the last 20 years, renal angioplasty and then stenting have replaced surgical treatment of RAS (Table 7.1). Stenting is favoured for the treatment of atherosclerotic RAS because such lesions often affect the ostium of the renal artery—an area where balloon angioplasty is complicated by late restenosis (Figure 7.7). This is an example of a technical procedure that has been endorsed by guidelines without any evidence, other than anecdotal, of survival benefits. The complications of stenting include arterial puncture problems and contrast reactions, but more serious adverse events can occur, including dissection and rupture of the renal artery. Stenting carries a small but definite procedural mortality risk. Technical failure may also be complicated by distal cholesterol embolization. A unique complication of technical success is of hypotension due to profound diuresis that can be avoided by careful attention to hydration status, and avoidance of antihypertensive drug therapy on the day of the procedure, although low-dose nifedipine is widely used as a peri-procedure therapy to reduce renal arterial spasm during manipulation.

A few small-scale studies have been confounded by a background of changing technology (surgery, angioplasty, stent, statins and available antihypertensive agents). The ASTRAL (Angioplasty and Stent for Renal Artery Lesions) trial, a large-scale UK-based study, randomized patients with atherosclerotic RAS where clinical uncertainty existed as to whether revascularization was indicated, to medical therapy or stenting. Preliminary reports suggest that there is no benefit of renal artery stenting compared with medical therapy

Table 7.1 Recommendations for treatment prior to ASTRAL trial

Patient characteristics	Treatment
Controlled blood pressure Minimal renal impairment (eGFR > 60) Renal artery stenosis (<50%) (unilateral or bilateral)	Medical
Advanced renal failure and small kidneys (<8 cm) and/or Renal artery occlusion (without distal recanalization) and/or No evidence of renal function in affected kidney	No prospect of recovery with intervention
Renal size >8 cm and renal artery stenosis >50% and Poorly controlled blood pressure despite intensive medical therapy or Deterioration in renal function with angiotensin-converting enzyme or Progressive renal failure	Angioplasty plus stent

eGFR = estimated glomerular filtration rate.

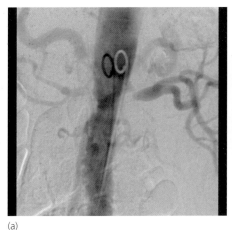
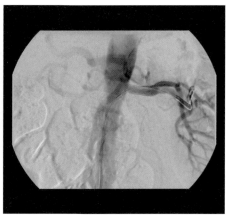

(a)   (b)

Figure 7.7 Endovascular treatment. Tight left renal artery stenosis before (a) and after (b) successful angioplasty and stenting, with an excellent morphological result achieved

Table 7.2 Clinical trials in renal artery stenosis

Trial	Number of patients	Intervention	End-point	Outcome
ASTRAL	806	Stenting vs medical therapy	Rate of decline of 1/creatinine over 1 year+	No difference in creatinine, blood pressure or vascular events in stent compared with medical therapy
NITER	~100	Stenting vs medical therapy	Death, dialysis or >20% of eGFR over 2 years	Report 2008–2009
CORAL	~1080	Stenting with embolic protection vs medical therapy	Death, cardiovascular event or dialysis	Recruiting
Van de Ven et al.	94	Angioplasty with and without stent placement	Degree of stenosis at 6 months	RAS stenosis rate 36% lower in stent group
Van Jaarsveld et al. (DRASTIC)	106	Angioplasty vs medical therapy	Blood pressure and renal function at 12 months	No difference between groups

in terms of decline of renal function, blood pressure or overall vascular events for the majority of patients with RAS (Table 7.2). This trial, and other similar trials, will shape the management of RAS in the future. At present, with increased appreciation of the complications of stenting and uncertainty over the benefits on blood pressure or renal function, vascular intervention is best reserved for patients with RAS and severe, resistant hypertension, patients with rapidly deteriorating renal function, or individuals with cardiorenal failure.

Further reading

Balk E, Raman G, Chung M *et al.* Effectiveness of management strategies for renal artery stenosis: a systematic review. *Ann Intern Med* 2006;**145**:901–1112.

Brady AJ, Mackenzie IS, Ritchie S *et al.* Grand rounds at the British Hypertension Society: renal artery stenosis. *J Hum Hypertens* 2007;**21**:750–755.

Conlon PJ, Athirakul K, Kovalik E *et al.* Survival in renal vascular disease. *J Am Soc Nephrol* 1998;**9**:252–256.

Ives NJ, Wheatley K, Stowe RL *et al.* Continuing uncertainty about the value of percutaneous revascularization in atherosclerotic renovascular disease: a meta-analysis of randomized trials. *Nephrol Dial Transplant* 2003;**18**:298–304.

Kalra PA, Guo H, Kausz AT *et al.* Atherosclerotic renovascular disease in United States patients aged 67 years or older: risk factors, revascularization, and prognosis. *Kidney Int* 2005;**68**:293–301.

McLaughlin K, Jardine AG, Moss JG. ABC of arterial and venous disease. Renal artery stenosis. *BMJ* 2000;**320**:1124–1127.

Mistry S, Ives N, Harding J, Fitzpatrick-Ellis K *et al.* Angioplasty and STent for Renal Artery Lesions (ASTRAL trial): rationale, methods and results so far. *J Hum Hypertens* 2007;**21**:511–515.

Murphy TP, Cooper CJ, Dworkin LD *et al.* The cardiovascular outcomes with renal atherosclerotic lesions (CORAL) study: rationale and methods. *J Vasc Interv Radiol* 2005;**16**:1295–1300.

Scarpioni R, Michieletti E, Cristinelli L *et al.* Atherosclerotic renovascular disease: medical therapy versus medical therapy plus renal artery stenting in preventing renal failure progression: the rationale and study design of a prospective, multicenter and randomized trial (NITER). *J Nephrol* 2005;**18**:423–428.

Siddiqui S, MacGregor MS, Glynn C *et al.* Factors predicting outcome in a cohort of patients with atherosclerotic renal artery disease diagnosed by magnetic resonance angiography. *Am J Kidney Dis* 2005;**46**:1065–1073.

Textor SC. Pitfalls in imaging for renal artery stenosis. *Ann Intern Med* 2004;**141**:730–731.

Uder M, Humke U. Endovascular therapy of renal artery stenosis: where do we stand today? *Cardiovasc Intervent Radiol* 2005;**28**:139–147.

van de Ven PJ, Kaatee R, Beutler JJ *et al.* Arterial stenting and balloon angioplasty in ostial atherosclerotic renovascular disease: a randomised trial. *Lancet* 1999;**353**:282–286.

van Jaarsveld BC, Krijnen P, Pieterman H *et al.* The effect of balloon angioplasty on hypertension in atherosclerotic renal artery stenosis. Dutch Renal Artery Stenosis Intervention Cooperative Study Group. *N Engl J Med* 2000;**342**:1007–1014.

Vasbinder GB, Nelemans PJ, Kessels AG *et al.* Renal Artery Diagnostic Imaging Study in Hypertension (RADISH) Study Group. Accuracy of computed tomographic angiography and magnetic resonance angiography for diagnosing renal artery stenosis. *Ann Intern Med* 2004;**141**:674–682.

Zalunardo N, Tuttle KR. Atherosclerotic renal artery stenosis: current status and future directions. *Curr Opin Nephrol Hypertens* 2004:**13**:613–621.

CHAPTER 8

Abdominal Aortic Aneurysms

Matthew J Bown, Guy Fishwick, Robert D Sayers

OVERVIEW

- The infrarenal abdominal aorta is the most common site for arterial aneurysm.
- Abdominal aortic aneurysms (AAAs) cause ~10 000 deaths per annum in England and Wales. The overall community mortality from ruptured AAAs is nearly 90%.
- Smoking is the most significant risk factor for AAA. The prevalence of AAA is nearly 6-fold greater in males than in females.
- Despite convincing studies proving the benefits of ultrasound screening for AAA, no national screening programme exists in the UK at present.
- The peri-operative mortality of endovascular repair is one-third of that of open repair, and this benefit in reduced risk from AAA related death is borne out long-term.

Introduction

The infrarenal abdominal aorta is the most common site for arterial aneurysms, the vast majority of which are fusiform in shape (Figure 8.1). Abdominal aortic aneurysms (AAAs) cause ~10 000 deaths per annum in England and Wales, and in 2003 were the eighth most common cause of death. In addition, deaths due to ruptured AAAs have nearly doubled over recent years (Figure 8.2) and this increase has been largely amongst the elderly ($\geq$80 years old) population.

Definition

The definition of aneurysmal arterial dilatation is an increase in vessel diameter of $\geq$50% in relation to an adjacent normal arterial segment. For practical purposes (in the case of the abdominal aorta) a measurement of >3 cm in any axial diameter is taken to be diagnostic for AAA. Normal infrarenal diameter is 2–2.4 cm in males and 1.6–2.2 cm in females.

Prevalence

In population screening studies of men, estimates for prevalence of AAAs >3 cm in size vary from 5 to 8.4%. The prevalence of AAA is lower in women at ~1.5%. AAA is a disease of Western nations; they are extremely rare in Asian populations and this appears to be a genetic effect as Asian populations in the UK have a much lower incidence of AAA than UK Caucasians.

Risk factors for abdominal aortic aneurysm (Box 8.1)

Smoking is the most significant risk factor for AAA, and this has been confirmed by several prospective studies which have also demonstrated a dose-dependent relationship with relative risk from 2.6 to 9.0 of AAA in smokers compared with non-smokers. The duration of smoking rather than amount smoked has a more significant effect on the risk of AAA formation, and the risk of AAA only gradually reduces over time after smoking cessation.

Other risk factors have been identified for the formation of AAA, although the strengths of these associations are not as well defined as for smoking. Hypertension has been associated with AAA in some studies, but other studies have failed to demonstrate this association. Similarly for hyperlipidaemia, some studies have demonstrated a positive association whilst others have not. Interestingly, diabetes mellitus has been shown to have either no association with AAA or even an inverse association. This inverse relationship may, however, be due to the high morbidity and mortality associated with diabetes mellitus preventing patients surviving to ages where AAA becomes prevalent.

Box 8.1 **Risk factors for AAA**

Proven
- Tobacco smoking
- Age >60 years
- Gender (males)

Possible
- Hypertension
- Hyperlipidaemia

ABC of Arterial & Venous Disease, 2nd edn. Edited by R. Donnelly and N. London.
© 2009 Blackwell Publishing Ltd. 9781405178891.

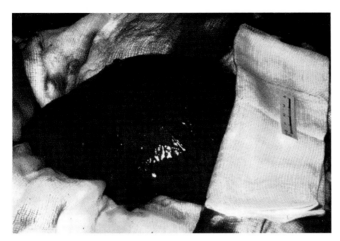

Figure 8.1 Operative photograph of an intact AAA

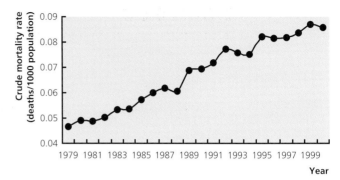

Figure 8.2 Death rates due to ruptured abdominal aortic aneurysm 1979–2000. Extracted from Series DH2 (5-26). *Mortality by cause*. The Stationery Office, London, 1980–2001

Non-environmental risk factors for AAA are age and gender. AAA rarely affects patients below the age of 40 years, and with increasing age the prevalence of AAA increases. Above the age of 65, each 7-year age increment confers a 1.5-fold increase in risk of AAA. AAA is predominately a disease of males, the prevalence being nearly 6-fold greater in males than females. The odds ratio for AAA formation in females is 0.2 compared with males.

Symptoms, signs and complications

The majority of AAAs (90%) are asymptomatic until the onset of complications, the most serious of which is rupture. Thin patients may notice a pulsatile swelling in their abdomen (Figure 8.3). The complications of any aneurysm are due to rupture, thrombosis or embolism. Acute thrombosis can occur in AAA but is more common at other aneurysmal sites such as the popliteal artery. Embolization of thrombus from AAA causing acute distal ischaemia (trash-foot) is more common than acute thrombosis (Figure 8.4). Together acute thrombosis or embolism only occur in 3–5% of patients with AAA.

The classical presenting triad of ruptured AAA (RAAA) is pain, either abdominal or back pain, hypotension and a pulsatile abdominal mass. Since only ~25% of patients with RAAA present with all three signs, a high index of suspicion for RAAA is essential in any patient who presents with any one of these symptoms and signs. Some patients may develop signs related to retroperitoneal haemorrhage such as flank or peri-umbilical bruising (Figure 8.5).

Diagnosis

Clinical examination is not a reliable tool for the diagnosis of AAA. The simplest diagnostic test for AAA is ultrasound, which has a sensitivity and specificity approaching 100%. This also has the advantage of not requiring ionizing radiation and, since ultrasound technology is portable, it lends itself to being used as a community screening tool. CT scanning has a similar sensitivity and specificity for the diagnosis of AAA to ultrasound. Additional information can be obtained regarding the morphology and anatomical relationships of the AAA (Figure 8.6). This is essential in planning surgery and determining suitability for endovascular repair. MRI provides similar information to CT but with the disadvantage of additional cost and limited patient acceptability. The main advantage of MRI

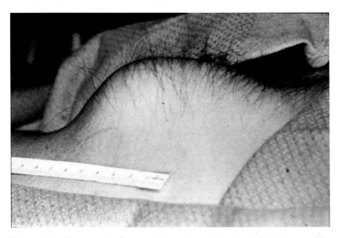

Figure 8.3 Photograph of a very thin patient with a large AAA that could be both seen and felt by the patient

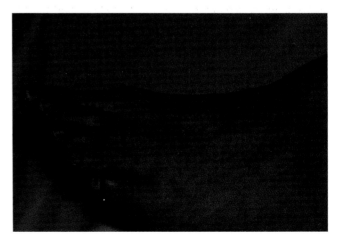

Figure 8.4 Focal infarction of areas of the first, second and third toes of the left foot in a patient with an AAA due to microembolization of thrombus from within the aneurysm sac (trash-foot)

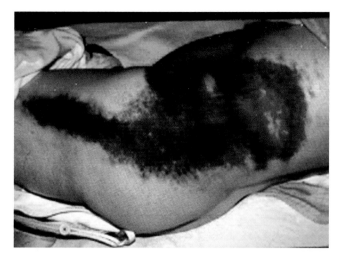

Figure 8.5 Flank bruising due to retroperitoneal blood from a ruptured AAA tracking laterally into the subcutaneous tissues. A rare sign of a ruptured AAA

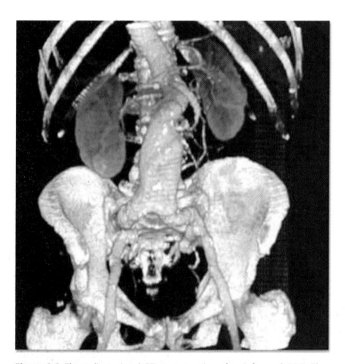

Figure 8.6 Three-dimensional CT reconstruction of an infrarenal AAA. The kidneys and bony skeleton have been included in the reconstruction for reference

is in the avoidance of ionizing radiation. Percutaneous aortography is of historical interest only.

In emergency situations, ultrasound scanning is useful to confirm the presence/absence of an AAA but cannot provide any information on the likelihood of AAA rupture. It is of most use in haemodynamically stable patients in whom the diagnosis of AAA is not suspected but needs to be excluded. CT scanning is both >90% sensitive and specific for the detection of ruptured AAA. Modern CT scanners can acquire images in as little as 30 s and thus cause little delay in transferring patients to theatre for surgery. The extra information provided and the possibility of assessment for endo-

vascular repair in centres where this service exists are of significant benefit.

Risk of rupture

Before surgery for AAA was developed in the second half of the 20th century, studies of patients with AAA who were left untreated demonstrated that 81.1% will die within 5 years compared with only 20.9% of the normal age-matched population. After 8 years only 10% of those with AAA are alive compared with 65% of the normal population. In patients with AAA unfit for surgery, a quarter will die due to AAA rupture, and the majority of these ruptures (80%) occur within 3 years of diagnosis.

AAA size is the single most important factor in determining the risk of rupture. Studies of ruptured AAA have demonstrated that the median size is usually >8 cm in diameter whereas only a very small proportion of screening-detected asymptomatic cases (0.16%) are >6 cm in diameter. Autopsy studies have found that RAAAs are significantly larger than incidentally found intact AAAs (8 cm vs 4 cm). This implies that aneurysms are at higher risk of rupture as they increase in size.

Patients with large aneurysms (>5.5 cm) are usually offered surgery providing they are fit enough. Patients with smaller aneurysms are a more difficult group to manage. In 1998 the results of the UK Small Aneurysm Trial were published. A total of 1090 patients with asymptomatic AAA between 4.0 and 5.5 cm were randomized to either surgery or surveillance with ultrasound scans every 3–6 months. After 4 years of follow-up there was no significant difference in mortality between the early surgery or surveillance groups. Since this trial, patients with asymptomatic AAA that are <5.5 cm are usually monitored ultrasonographically rather than offered surgery. Because of this relationship between size and risk of rupture, AAA size becomes the critical factor dictating clinical management.

Screening for AAA

The fact that AAAs are often asymptomatic until rupture, the high mortality associated with rupture and the availability of a sensitive and acceptable test for AAA raises the potential for screening asymptomatic patients for AAA. This concept has been addressed by the Multicentre Aneurysm Screening Study (MASS), reported in 2002. This study randomized 67 800 men between the ages of 65 and 74 years to ultrasound screening or not. In the control group there were 113 aneurysm-related deaths compared with only 65 in the screened group (42% risk reduction) and the projected 10-year cost per quality-adjusted life year (QALY) gained was only £8000. Currently, no national screening programme yet exists in the UK although the UK government has recently announced that one will be implemented in the near future.

Surveillance

Patients with a small AAA (<5.5 cm) are usually not offered surgery as the risks of surgery outweigh the risk of rupture. However, because it is known that small AAAs grow with time, it is important to provide surveillance for these patients. This is usually in the form of serial ultrasound scanning, and most centres scan smaller AAAs (3–4.5 cm) every 6–12 months and AAAs between 4.5 and 5.5 cm every 3–6 months.

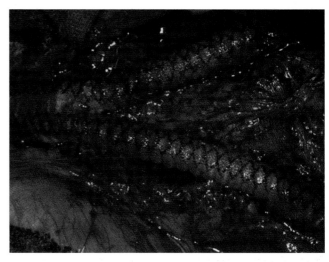

Figure 8.7 Operative photograph of a bifurcated Dacron graft inlay AAA repair. The proximal anastomosis lies beyond the left of the picture

Treatment

Currently the only curative treatment for AAA is surgery (Box 8.2). Traditionally this has consisted of open abdominal repair. However, since the early 1990s, endovascular techniques have become widely available and are rapidly advancing. Whilst AAA is the main focus of this chapter, it should not be forgotten that each patient is likely to have significant cardiovascular risk factors and there is the opportunity to address these and provide medical therapy such as antiplatelet agents and statins in all patients.

Elective AAA repair

The majority of patients with asymptomatic AAAs are diagnosed incidentally and considered for surgery if their AAA is >5.5 cm. Aside from an assessment of overall patient fitness, paying particular attention to cardiorespiratory and renal investigations, a CT scan is obtained to determine the anatomy of the AAA and suitability for endovascular repair.

Open AAA repair consists of a laparotomy, isolation of the aneurysmal aorta between vascular clamps and, after opening the aneurysm sac, suturing a synthetic graft in place and then closing the sac over the graft (an inlay repair) (Figure 8.7). This is a major procedure with a peri-operative mortality between 3 and 8% and a risk of major systemic complications of ~25%. Endovascular AAA repair is an alternative to open repair in those patients with anatomically suitable aneurysms (Figure 8.8). This procedure is much less invasive, requiring only small femoral artery cut-down incisions rather than a full laparotomy. A suitably sized stent-graft is inserted via the femoral arteries and positioned in the infrarenal

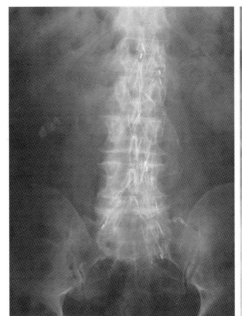
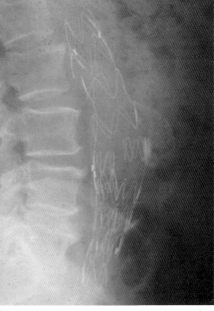

Figure 8.8 Plain (a) antero-posterior and (b) lateral abdominal radiographs showing an endovascular stent *in situ*. The calcified wall of the excluded aneurysm sac can be seen in both images, on the left in (a) and anteriorly in (b)

(a)   (b)

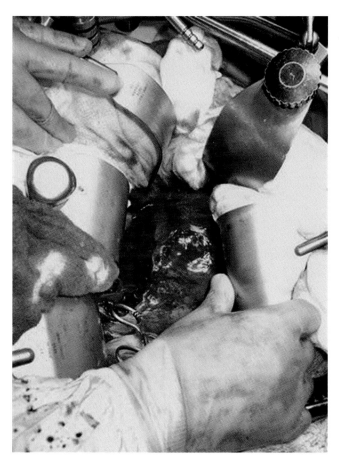

Figure 8.9 Operative photograph of a large retroperitoneal haematoma due to a ruptured AAA. The neck of the aneurysm is behind the haematoma at the top of the picture

aorta under radiological guidance using specialized delivery systems. This procedure has been shown to have a 3-fold lower peri-operative mortality than open repair in large randomized trials. This immediate survival advantage is offset by the requirement for long-term follow-up to detect potential complications that place the patient at continued risk of rupture—graft migra-

tion, graft material failure and leakage of blood around the graft into the AAA sac (endoleak). However, despite this, the immediate survival advantage of endovasular repair is borne out in the long term with an overall reduction in AAA related mortality at 4 years.

Ruptured AAA repair

The overall community mortality from a ruptured AAA is nearly 90%. In those patients who do reach hospital alive and undergo surgery (Figure 8.9), the peri-operative mortality is ~40%. Identifying those patients in whom surgery is futile is difficult. The most commonly used criteria predicting non-survival are extreme age (>80 years), pre-operative cardiac arrest, severe cardiorespiratory disease and unconsciousness.

Endovascular techniques have been used with limited success in the treatment of ruptured AAAs. Currently small case series have shown reduced peri-operative mortality rates compared with open repair using this technique, but to date there have been no randomized trials large enough to determine whether this is a beneficial alternative to open repair of ruptured AAA.

Further reading

Endovascular Aneurysm Repair: comparison of endovascular aneurysm repair with open repair in patients with abdominal aortic aneurysm (EVAR trial 1), 30-day operative mortality results: randomized controlled trial. The EVAR Trial Participants. *Lancet* 2004;**364**:843–848.

Multicentre Aneurysm Screening Study Group. Multicentre aneurysm screening study (MASS): cost effectiveness analysis of screening for abdominal aortic aneurysms based on four year results from randomized controlled trial. *BMJ* 2002;**325**:1135.

The UK Small Aneurysm Trial Participants. UK Small Aneurysm Trial: mortality results for randomized controlled trial of early elective surgery or ultrasonographic surveillance for small abdominal aortic aneurysms. *Lancet* 1998;**352**:1649–1655.

Endovascular aneurysm repair versus open repair in patients with abdominal aortic aneurysm (EVAR trial 1). The EVAR Trail Participants. *Lancet* 2005;**365**:2179–2186.

CHAPTER 9

Secondary Prevention of Peripheral Arterial Disease

Julie Brittenden

OVERVIEW

- Peripheral arterial disease (PAD) is an underdiagnosed and undertreated condition.

- PAD is a marker of underlying cardiovascular and cerebrovascular disease.

- In the REACH registry, patients with PAD had a higher mortality and cardiovascular event rates at 1 year compared with patients with cardiovascular disease.

- PAD patients with concomitant symptomatic cardiac or cerebrovascular disease or diabetes are at even higher risk of sustaining a vascular event.

- Secondary prevention for patients with PAD is the same as that for patients with coronary heart disease.

Introduction

Peripheral arterial disease (PAD) is common, with a prevalence of both symptomatic and asymptomatic disease estimated at 16% in the over 55 age group. Patients diagnosed as having PAD have widespread arterial disease and a 2- to 3-fold increased risk of cardiovascular and cerebrovascular mortality when compared with an age- and sex-matched group without PAD. The increased mortality is evident even in patients with asymptomatic disease and increases with the severity of disease (Figure 9.1). A 10-year study showed that patients with PAD affecting large vessels had a 6.6-fold (95% CI 2.9–14.9) increase in risk of death from coronary heart disease compared with patients with no PAD. In this study, less than a quarter of patients with severe symptomatic large vessel PAD survived 10 years (Figure 9.1).

The ABPI has, in addition to diagnosing PAD, been shown to predict overall survival. Significant linear trends have been shown across ABPI categories and cardiovascular outcome in a number of studies, which is independent of the metabolic syndrome and other conventional cardiovascular risk factors (Figure 9.2).

The current global Reduction of Atherothrombosis for Continued Health (REACH) registry, aims to evaluate atherothrombotic risk in >68 000 at-risk patients. To date, it has shown that compared with patients with cardiovascular and cerebrovascular disease, those with PAD had the highest death rates at 1 year (Figure 9.3). Furthermore, the incidence of cardiovascular death, myocardial infarction or stroke increased with the number of symptomatic arterial disease locations.

Cardiovascular risk factor management in PAD

Evidence-based medicine has shown that reducing cardiovascular risk in patients with symptomatic PAD improves survival. The major risk factors for both cardiovascular disease and PAD—cigarette smoking, dyslipidaemia, hypertension, diabetes and lifestyle issues—are well recognized, as is the need for antiplatelet therapy (Table 9.1). The rationale and targets for treating these risks factors have been addressed in a number of national and international guidelines including the recently updated and revised Scottish intercollegiate (SIGN) guidelines on the management of PAD and the Transatlantic Society (TASC) guidelines. The management of these risk factors is outlined below.

Dyslipidaemia

In 2002, the MRC Heart Protection study clearly demonstrated the benefits of statin therapy in patients with PAD. Treatment with simvastatin 40 mg daily resulted in a 22% (95% CI 15–29) relative risk reduction in the rates of myocardial infarction, stroke and of revascularization in patients with PAD who had a cholesterol level >3.5 mmol/l. There was also a significant reduction in all-cause mortality and in particular that due to cardiac causes in patients with PAD allocated to simvastatin therapy (Figure 9.4). Current recommendations are that patients with intermittent claudication (IC) with a total cholesterol >3.5 mmol/l should be commenced on statin therapy (Table 9.1).

The reduction in vascular events achieved by statin therapy is greater than would be predicted from the lipid-lowering effects alone. In the heart protection study, the reduction in major vascular events was evident following 1 year of treatment, whereas other

ABC of Arterial & Venous Disease, 2nd edn. Edited by R. Donnelly and N. London.
© 2009 Blackwell Publishing Ltd. 9781405178891.

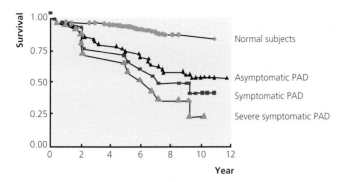

Figure 9.1 Kaplan–Meier survival curves based on mortality from all causes in patients with large vessel disease. PAD = peripheral artery disease. Produced from Criqui *et al.* (1992)

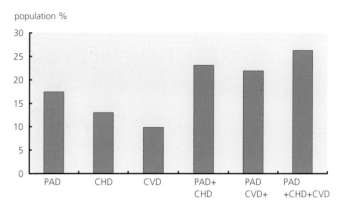

Figure 9.3 One-year cardiovascular event rates in outpatients with atherothrombosis. PAD = peripheral vascular disease; CHD = coronary heart disease; CVD = cerebrovascular disease. Data for the graph were obtained from Steg *et al.* (2007)

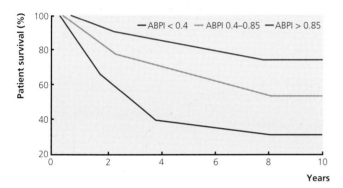

Figure 9.2 The ratio of ankle and arm arterial pressure as an independent predictor of mortality. McKenna *et al.* (1991)

non-statin therapies that lower LDL-cholesterol require up to 5 years to show a clinical effect. This had led to a debate over the exact mode of action of statins, in particular the relative contributions of their lipid- and non-lipid- (isoprenoid) lowering properties to cardiac risk prevention (Figures 9.5 and 9.6). While variations may exist between statins and their so-called pleiotropic effects,

insufficient data exist to allow us to determine which is the most effective statin. Furthermore, the cholesterol-lowering effects should not be underestimated.

A prospective meta-analysis of 14 randomized trials of statins has shown that the reductions in cardiovascular risk were proportional to the achieved absolute LDL-cholesterol reduction (Figure 9.7). Overall, statins reduced the 5-year incidence of major coronary events, coronary revascularization and stroke by one-fifth per mmol/l reduction in LDL-cholesterol, irrespective of the patient's baseline lipid profile. Thus, it is not merely sufficient to start the patient with PAD on a statin without closely monitoring their level of cholesterol reduction. Furthermore, recent trials involving patients with acute coronary syndromes and stable coronary disease have shown a greater reduction in cardiac events in patients receiving high-dose compared with conventional dose statin therapy. This is likely to be the case for patients with PAD and perhaps should be considered for those most at risk, such as those with

Table 9.1 Cardiovascular risk factor management in patients with PAD

Risk factor	Treatment
Antiplatelet	All patients should be commenced on antiplatelet therapy
Dyslipidaemia	Start statin therapy if cholesterol level is >3.5 mmol/l Monitor to assess reduction in cholesterol
Hypertension	Commence antihypertensive therapy in order to achieve the following targets: In people without diabetes Maintain below 140/85 mmHg In people with diabetes Maintain below 130/80 mmHg
Diabetes	Screen for diabetes Aggressively treat to lower glycosylated haemogloblin to <7%
Smoking	Actively encourage patient to stop smoking In willing patients: refer to smoking cessation councillor/therapy, prescribe nicotine replacement therapy Consider bupropion (zyban), varenicline tartrate (champix)
Lifestyle issues	Advise regular exercise Obese patients should be treated to reduce their weight

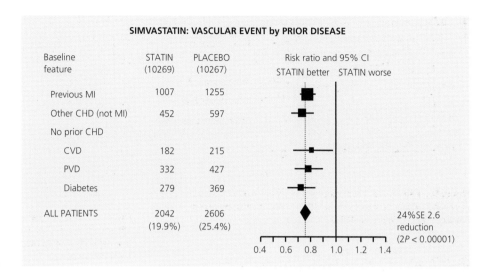

Figure 9.4 Heart protection study. Heart Protection Study Collaborative Group (2002)

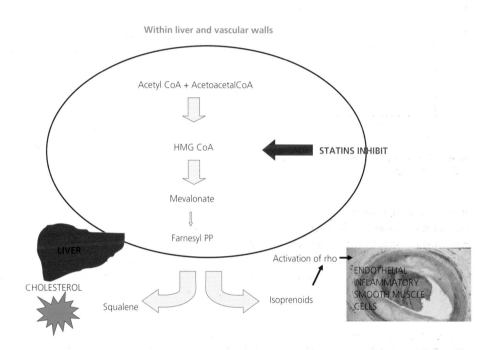

Figure 9.5 Mode of action of statins

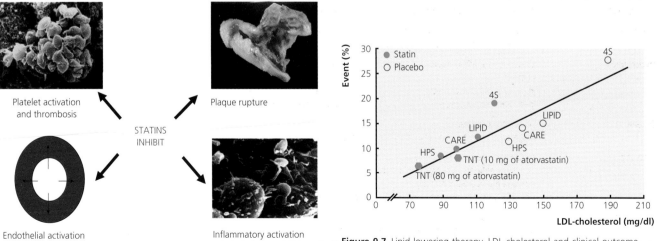

Figure 9.6 Pleiotropic effects of statins

Figure 9.7 Lipid lowering therapy, LDL-cholesterol and clinical outcome. Produced from La Rosa et al. (2005)

concurrent diabetes and a low ABPI. However, the cost-effectiveness of such a strategy is not yet known.

Most other lipid-lowering therapies have been superseded by statins. Dietary measures may reduce serum cholesterol and LDL-cholesterol by 10%, but long-term compliance is low (Box 9.1).

Box 9.1 **Statin therapy**

Statins reduce the rates of myocardial infarction, stroke and revascularization in patients with PAD
• Irrespective of the baseline cholesterol
• In proportion to the achieved reduction in LDL-cholesterol

Blood pressure

Elevated blood pressure is an independent risk factor for cardio-vascular and cerebrovascular morbidity and mortality. In the Framingham trial, the age-adjusted risk ratio for IC in hypertensive patients compared with controls was increased 2.5- to 4-fold. In patients with T2DM and PAD, intensive blood pressure control has been shown to reduce the risk of cardiovascular events significantly. The current British hypertensive society guidelines recommend a target level of <140/90 mmHg or 130/80 mmHg for diabetics or patients with chronic renal disease, respectively. While β-blockers are no longer the recommended first-line treatment for hypertension, their use in patients with PAD has not been shown to worsen the symptoms of claudication according to a meta-analysis of 11 randomized controlled trials. Furthermore, with the ready availability of non-vasoconstrictor β-blockers this treatment option should not be withheld from patients with PAD.

ACE inhibitors can be safely used to treat hypertension in patients with PAD but should be commenced with careful monitoring. The incidence of RAS in the PAD population as a whole is difficult to ascertain, but may be present in a quarter of patients with PAD undergoing angiography. Since the publication of the Heart Outcomes Prevention Evaluation (HOPE) study, there has been a move towards recommending the use of ACE inhibitors in patients with PAD even in the absence of hypertension. ACE inhibitors have been shown to have various pleiotropic effects beyond their blood pressure-lowering capacity. While there appears to be a promising reduction in cardiovascular mortality, morbidity and stroke associated with ACE inhibitors, not all guidelines recommend their use in patients with PAD. While it is apparent that the beneficial effects were seen in patients with clinical and subclinical evidence of PAD as assessed by ABPI using palpation of pedal pulses, it is unclear if this occurred equally in 'non-hypertensive' and 'hypertensive' patients. Furthermore, only 30% of patients in the HOPE study were on statin therapy, and thus the pleiotropic effects of ACE inhibitors in addition to standard medical therapy in patients with PAD requires to be evaluated further.

Glycaemic control

Diabetes and its poor control have long been recognized as a major risk factor for PAD. In the Framingham trial, the age-adjusted risk

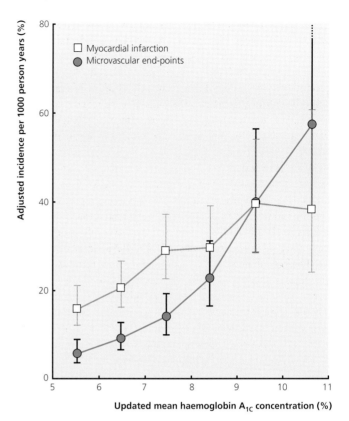

Figure 9.8 Diabetes, HbA$_{1c}$ and macrovascular events. Produced from Stratton *et al.* (2000)

ratio for IC in diabetic patients compared with controls was five times greater for men and four times greater for women.

Even amongst new referrals to a vascular clinic, undiagnosed diabetes is common, occurring in at least 12% of patients. Furthermore, although diabetic patients make up ~20% of the PAD population, 80% of amputations are in this group. Tight diabetic control has been shown to reduce the risk of developing microvascular and macrovascular complications. The UK diabetes prospective observation study analysis found that over a 10-year period, each 1% reduction in HbA$_{1c}$ has been shown to correlate with a 14% reduction in myocardial infarction and a 43% decrease in amputation or death from PAD (Figure 9.8).

Antiplatelet therapy

Antiplatelet therapy protects against non-fatal myocardial infarction, non-fatal stroke and vascular death in patients with IC. Overall in patients with PAD, antiplatelet therapy has been shown to result in a 23% reduction in these events. The Antithrombotic Trialist collaboration found no differences between aspirin, ticlopidine and dipyridamole. Evidence shows that low-dose aspirin (75–150 mg) is equally as effective as high doses and is associated with a lower rate of gastrointestinal side effects. The SIGN guidelines recommend the use of antiplatelet therapy, but do not stipulate which antiplatelet agent should be used as first-line therapy.

The clopidogrel versus aspirin in patients at high risk of ischaemic events trial (CAPRIE) showed that clopidogrel reduced the relative risk of major vascular events by 8.7% (95% CI 0.3–16.5%) compared with aspirin. In a subgroup analysis, clopidogrel reduced the relative risk of major vascular events by 23.8% (95% CI 8.9–36.2%) compared with aspirin in patients with PAD. A subsequent economic analysis by NICE has shown that the use of clopidogrel as first-line antiplatelet therapy exceeds their target cost per QALY and thus it is not considered to be cost-effective. It remains to be determined if clopidogrel is cost-effective in the 'higher risk' PAD groups.

Platelet activation despite the use of aspirin therapy has been shown to be increased in patients with PAD compared with healthy controls. The incidence of 'non-responsiveness' to aspirin increases with the severity of disease and following major revascularization surgery. It is difficult to ascertain the level of aspirin non-responsiveness in patients with PAD, and debate exists as to how this should be defined and measured. Data from our own laboratory suggest that this aspirin non-responsiveness may occur in 11–15% of patients with stable PAD and this may increase to almost 50% following surgery. Similarly, a large variation in response to clopidogrel has also been shown to occur in patients with IC, with up to 10% of patients showing no reduction in platelet activation after a loading dose (Box 9.2).

Box 9.2 **Antiplatelet therapy**

Antiplatelet therapy reduces the risk of myocardial infarction, stroke and vascular death in patients with PAD
- Clopidogrel is more effective than aspirin
- Combination therapy (aspirin and clopidogrel) is not more effective

---

Smoking

In the Framingham study, cigarette smoking increased the risk of developing IC by 2-fold. The cardiovascular health study showed that smoking resulted in a 2-fold increase in the progression of PAD.

In patients with PAD, cessation of smoking is associated with a 2-fold increase in their survival rate compared with patients who continue to smoke. While there is a lack of data regarding the efficacy of smoking cessation programmes in patients with PAD, it is likely to have the same benefits as for those with coronary heart disease.

Smoking cessation reduces the risk of mortality in patients with coronary heart disease, and benefits are observed within 1 year of stopping smoking. A recent Cochrane Review of smoking cessation for the secondary prevention of coronary heart disease has shown that smoking cessation is associated with a 36% reduction in all-cause mortality, which is much higher than that obtained from statin therapy. Encouraging patients to stop smoking through smoking cessation support programmes has been shown to double the smoking cessation rate. Similarly, nicotine replacement therapy increases the quit rate by ~2-fold. Antidepressants (bupropion and nortriptyline) have also been found useful in helping patients to stop smoking. Recently, it has been shown in a randomized controlled trial that patients taking varenicline had four times greater odds of stopping smoking compared with those on placebo and twice greater odds than those on bupropion (Box 9.3).

Box 9.3 **Smoking**

Smoking cessation is associated with a 36% reduction in all-cause mortality

---

Lifestyle: weight reduction and exercise

Obesity, in particular a body mass index (BMI) >30 kg/m^2, is associated with increased cardiovascular risk. Thus as part of general lifestyle measures, obese patients should be offered help with weight reduction. All patients should also be encouraged to exercise, but self-motivation to comply with unsupervised programmes may be an issue. Current studies in patients with PAD have assessed the effect of exercise on walking distance rather than cardiovascular outcome.

Homocysteine lowering

Hyperhomocysteinaemia is an independent risk factor for atherosclerosis and may be present in 50–60% of patients with PAD. It may be treated by folic acid and vitamin B$_6$ supplements. While homocysteine may be implicated in the progression of disease, there is currently no convincing evidence that treatment in patients with IC will alter the natural history of the disease. Thus routine measurement and treatment of homocysteine is currently not recommended.

Extent of risk factor management in patients with PAD

Recent surveys have demonstrated that secondary prevention of PAD in patients is suboptimal in primary and secondary care. In particular, in both the primary and secondary care setting, patients with PAD receive less intensive treatment for lipid disorders and hypertension and were prescribed antiplatelet therapy less frequently than were patients with coronary heart disease. It is thus unfortunate that in the UK patients with PAD are not targeted for secondary prevention therapy within primary care in the same manner as those with cardiovascular and cerebrovascular disease who have lesser risk profiles. In addition to being an undertreated disease, PAD is often underdiagnosed, and public awareness of the condition has been shown to be poor. This lack of awareness and suboptimal therapy urgently needs to be addressed (Box 9.4).

Box 9.4 **PAD**

PAD is a common condition that is underdiagnosed and is:
- Associated with a 2- to 3-fold increase in cardiovascular mortality
- Suboptimally managed in terms of risk factor prevention compared with coronary heart disease

Further reading

Antithrombotic Trialist Collaboration. Collaborative meta-analysis of randomized trials of antiplatelet therapy for the prevention of death, myocardial infarction and stroke in high risk patients. *BMJ* 2002;**324**:71–86.

Baigent C, Keech A, Keaney PM *et al*. Efficacy and safety of cholesterol-lowering treatment: prospective meta-analysis of data from 90,056 participants in 14 randomized trials of statins. *Lancet* 2005;**366**:1267–1278.

Belch JJF, Topol EH, Agnelli C *et al*. Critical issues in peripheral arterial disease detection and management: a call to action. *Arch Intern Med* 2003;**163**:884–892.

Burns P, Gough S, Bradbury AW. Management of peripheral arterial disease in primary care. *BMJ* 2003;**326**:584–588.

CAPRIE Steering Committee. A randomized, blinded, trial of clopidogrel versus aspirin in patients at risk of ischaemic events (CAPRIE). *Lancet* 1996;**348**:1329–1339.

Cassar K, Coull R, Bachoo P *et al*. Primary care risk factor management in claudicants. *Eur J Vasc Endovasc Surg* 2003;**26**:145–149.

Criqui MH, Langer RD, Fronek A *et al*. Mortality over a period of 10 years in patients with peripheral arterial disease. *N Engl J Med* 1992;**326**:381–386.

Critical Leg Ischaemia Prevention Study (CLIPS) Group. Prevention of serious vascular events by aspirin amongst patients with peripheral arterial disease: randomized, double-blind trial. *J Intern Med* 2007;**261**:276–284.

Fowkes FG, Housley E, Cawood EH *et al*. Edinburgh Artery Study: prevalence of asymptomatic and symptomatic peripheral arterial disease in the general population. *Int J Epidemiol* 1991;**20**:384–392.

Gasse C, Jacobsen J, Larsen AC *et al*. Secondary medical prevention among Danish patients hospitalized with either peripheral arterial disease or myocardial infarction. *Eur J Vasc Endovasc Surg* 2007;**35**:51–58.

Heart Outcomes Prevention Evaluation Study Investigators. Effects of angiotensin-converting enzyme inhibitor, ramipril, on cardiovascular events in high risk patients. *N Engl J Med* 2000;**342**:145–153.

Heart Protection Study Collaborative Group. MRC/BHF Heart Protection Study of cholesterol lowering with simvastatin in 20,536 high risk individuals: a randomized placebo controlled trail. *Lancet* 2002;**360**:7–22.

Hirsch AT, Criqui MH, Treat-Jacobson D *et al*. Peripheral arterial disease detection, awareness, and treatment in primary care. *JAMA* 2001;**286**:1317–1324.

Hirsch AT, Gotto AM Jr. Undertreatment of dyslipidaemia in peripheral arterial disease and other high risk populations: an opportunity for cardiovascular disease reduction. *Vasc Med* 2002;**7**:323–331.

LaRosa JC, Grundy SM, Walters DD *et al*. Intensive lipid lowering with atorvastatin in patients with stable coronary heart disease. *N Engl J Med* 2005;**352**:1425–1435.

Lee AJ, Price JF, Russell MJ *et al*. Improved prediction of fatal myocardial infarction using the ankle brachial index in addition to conventional risk factors: the Edinburgh Artery Study. *Circulation* 2004;**110**:3075–3080.

McKenna M, Wolfson S, Kuller L. The ratio of ankle and arm arterial pressure as an independent predictor of mortality. *Atherosclerosis* 1991;**87**:119–128.

Mohler ER. Peripheral arterial disease: identification and implications. *Arch Intern Med* 2003;**163**:2306–2314.

Scottish Intercollegiate Guidelines Network (SIGN). Diagnosis and management of peripheral arterial disease. 2006;**89**:12.

Steg PH, Bhatt D, Wilson PWF *et al*. One-year cardiovascular event rates in outpatients with atherothrombosis. *JAMA* 2007;**297**:1197–1206.

Stratton IM, Adler AI, Neil HAW *et al*. Association of macrovascular and microvascular complications of type 2 diabetes (UKPDS:35): prospective observational study. *BMJ* 2000;**321**:505–512.

TASC II guidelines at http://www.tasc-2-pad.org

CHAPTER 10

Vasculitis

Matthew D Morgan, Stuart W Smith, Caroline OS Savage

OVERVIEW

- The vasculitides are classified as primary or secondary, localized or systemic, and characterized by inflammation of blood vessels. The primary systemic vasculitides (PSVs) are usually grouped together as large, medium or small vessel diseases according to the smallest size of vessel involved.

- The mainstay of treatment for most PSV is still immunosuppression with corticosteroids and cytotoxic agents, but these drugs often cause significant morbidity.

- Giant cell arteritis is the most commont form of PSV in the UK, whereas Takayasu's arteritis is the most common in Asia.

- Polyarteritis nodosa (PAN) is uncommon in the UK, a disease of medium-sized arteries that leads to ischaemia or infarction within affected organs. Diagnosis is based on the demonstration of arterial aneurysms in the renal, splanchnic, hepatic or splenic vessels using angiography.

- For non-hepatitis B-associated PAN, the severity of disease at presentation predicts the long-term outcome, with poorer survival seen in those patients having more severe disease.

- The most serious feature of Kawasaki disease is coronary artery disease; aneurysms occur in a fifth of untreated patients and may lead to myocardial infarction.

- Small vessel vasculitis associated with antineutrophil cytoplasmic antibodies (ANCAs) may present with nonspecific symptoms, e.g. fever, malaise, arthralgia, myalgia and weight loss. Once respiratory or renal disease develops, the course is usually rapidly progressive.

- Wegener's granulomatosis, microscopic polyangiitis and Churg–Strauss syndrome have distinct features.

- Henoch–Schönlein purpura is mainly a disease of children and is usually self-limiting, requiring nothing more than supportive care. The typical features comprise purpura over the buttocks and lower limbs, haematuria, abdominal pain, bloody diarrhoea and arthralgia.

The vasculitides are a group of diseases causing inflammation in blood vessel walls. They are usually classified as primary or secondary (to diseases such as bacterial endocarditis, systemic lupus erythematosus or drugs such as propylthiouracil) and can be localized (affecting usually only the skin or a single organ system) or systemic (affecting multiple organ systems). This chapter will focus on the primary systemic vasculitides (PSVs). The PSVs are usually grouped together as large, medium or small vessel diseases according to the smallest size of vessel involved (Figure 10.1).

The aetiopathogenesis is still not well understood for most PSVs, and so the classification of the diseases is not completely satisfactory. Most PSVs have classification criteria that were defined at the Chapel Hill Consensus Conference (CHCC). These classification criteria are based on a combination of clinical features and pathological findings. The CHCC classification criteria will be used throughout this chapter.

The clinical features seen in PSVs can be divided into those features that are common to most systemic inflammatory diseases (fever, malaise, weight loss, night sweats, arthralgia and myalgia) and those features that are specific to the organ systems involved in the disease. Evidence of an acute phase response is common to most active PSVs, with a raised serum C-reactive protein (CRP) and erythrocyte sedimentation rate (ESR) or plasma viscosity (PV).

Because the pathogenesis is still poorly understood, the mainstay of treatment for most PSVs is still immunosuppression with corticosteroids and cytotoxic agents. Many of the immunosuppressive regimes used in PSVs are associated with considerable morbidity and mortality. Many of the drug trials in recent years have been designed to investigate therapeutic regimes which reduce the immunosuppressive burden for patients whilst still maintaining disease control.

Large vessel vasculitis

Giant cell arteritis (temporal arteritis)

Giant cell arteritis is the most common form of PSV in the UK. It may affect any of the major branches of the aorta. Clinical features include unilateral throbbing headache, facial pain and claudication of the jaw when eating (Box 10.1). Visual loss is a feared

ABC of Arterial & Venous Disease, 2nd edn. Edited by R. Donnelly and N. London. © 2009 Blackwell Publishing Ltd. 9781405178891.

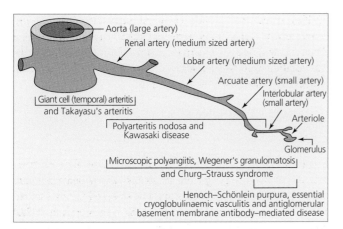

Figure 10.1 Spectrum of systemic vasculitides organized according to predominant size of vessels affected (adopted from Jennette *et al.*, 1992)

> Box 10.1 **Definitions of large vessel vasculitis**
>
> **Giant cell arteritis (temporal arteritis)**
> - Granulomatous arteritis of aorta and its major branches, especially extracranial branches of carotid artery
> - Often affects temporal artery
> - Usually occurs in patients older than 50 years
> - Often associated with polymyalgia rheumatica
>
> **Takayasu's arteritis**
> - Granulomatous inflammation of aorta and its major branches
> - Usually occurs in patients younger than 50 years

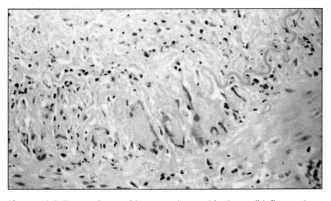

Figure 10.2 Temporal artery biopsy specimen with giant cell inflammation

complication of the disease, and it may be sudden and painless, affecting some or all of the visual field. Diplopia and other cranial nerve lesions may occur.

Initial treatment is with high dose prednisolone (40–60 mg/day), which should be started as soon as the diagnosis is suspected to avoid visual loss. The diagnosis is confirmed by biopsy of the affected artery (Figure 10.2). The addition of methylprednisolone may improve remission rates and reduce corticosteroid exposure. Recent studies have investigated the use of MRI and positron emission tomography (PET) in the initial assessment of disease extent and monitoring of vascular inflammation. The corticosteroid dose

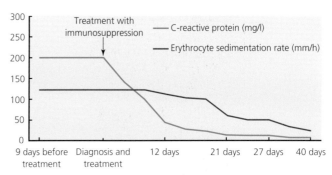

Figure 10.3 C-reactive protein concentration (>10 mg/l) and erythrocyte sedimentation rate (>18 mm/h) are raised at time of diagnosis of giant cell arteritis but fall to normal levels after starting immunosuppression therapy

may be reduced to 10 mg/day over 6 months and then more slowly to a maintenance of 5–10 mg/day. Maintenance treatment may be required for 2 years. The addition of methotrexate to corticosteroids may reduce relapse risk, as well as corticosteroid exposure. Etanercept may allow a reduction of corticosteroid dose for patients with side effects. Prevention of platelet aggregation with low-dose aspirin is potentially effective in preventing ischaemic complications of GCA. The disease is monitored by measuring acute phase response markers and sometimes using non-invasive imaging (Figure 10.3).

Takayasu's arteritis

Takayasu's arteritis (Box 10.1) is most common in Asia, affects more women than men and is usually diagnosed in patients <50 years of age. Inflammation and then scarring of the aorta and its major branches leads to aortic arch syndrome with claudication of the arm, loss of pulses, variation of blood pressure of >10 mmHg between the arms, arterial bruits, angina, aortic valve regurgitation, syncope, stroke and visual disturbance. Involvement of the descending aorta may cause bowel ischaemia, mesenteric angina, renovascular hypertension, renal impairment and lower limb claudication.

Diagnosis is by angiography, MRI or PET scanning. Treatment of acute disease in patients with high CRP or ESR is with corticosteroids. Cytotoxic drugs such as cyclophosphamide can be added if steroids alone do not control the disease. Surgery or angioplasty may be required for stenoses once active inflammation has been controlled.

Medium vessel vasculitis

Polyarteritis nodosa

Polyarteritis nodosa (Box 10.2) is uncommon in the UK. It is associated with hepatitis B virus (HBV) infection in some patients. Disease of medium-sized arteries leads to ischaemia or infarction within affected organs. The disease can involve the gut, causing abdominal pain, bleeding or perforation; in the heart it can cause angina or myocardial infarction; cortical infarcts and ischaemia in the kidneys can lead to renal impairment and hypertension; and involvement of the peripheral nervous system can cause mononeuritis multiplex.

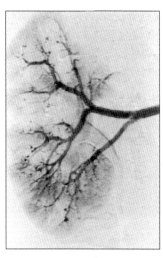

Figure 10.4 Renal angiogram showing multiple arterial aneurysms

Diagnosis is based on the demonstration of arterial aneurysms in the renal, splanchnic, hepatic or splenic vessels using angiography (Figure 10.4). Biopsy of affected muscles or nerves may reveal histological evidence of arteritis.

Treatment of polyarteritis associated with HBV requires an antiviral drug such as interferon α or Lamivudine combined with short-course, high-dose corticosteroids and plasma exchange. For non-HBV-associated PAN, the severity of disease at presentation predicts the long-term outcome, with poorer survival seen in those patients having more severe disease. The addition of cyclophosphamide to corticosteroids for 12 months may improve outcomes for patients with severe disease.

Kawasaki disease

Kawasaki disease (Box 10.2) usually affects children under the age of 12 years. The typical clinical features are described in Box 10.3. The most serious feature of Kawasaki disease is coronary artery disease; aneurysms occur in a fifth of untreated patients and may lead to myocardial infarction. They can be detected by echocardiography and, in severe circumstances, coronary reperfusion strategies are required. High-dose intravenous immunoglobulins (IVIGs) reduce the prevalence of coronary artery aneurysms, provided that treatment is started within 10 days of onset of the disease. Low-dose aspirin is recommended for thrombocythaemia. The addition of corticosteroids to aspirin and IVIG may reduce the incidence of coronary artery aneurysms.

Small vessel vasculitis associated with antineutrophil cytoplasmic antibodies

The early symptoms of these disorders are nonspecific, with fever, malaise, arthralgia, myalgia and weight loss, and patients in whom such symptoms are persistent should be screened for antineutrophil cytoplasmic antibodies (ANCAs), have their ESR and CRP concentration measured and have their urine tested for blood with a dipstick. Early diagnosis is essential to prevent potentially life-threatening renal and pulmonary injury. Delays in diagnosis are unfortunately common, and this often leads to serious morbidity. Once respiratory or renal disease develops, the course is usually rapidly progressive.

Wegener's granulomatosis

Upper respiratory tract disease occurs in >90% of cases. Limited Wegener's refers to disease that affects only the respiratory tract at the time of diagnosis; many cases evolve to systemic disease. Lung disease is common, with cough, haemoptysis and dyspnoea, and may progress to life-threatening pulmonary haemorrhage. The kidneys are affected in up to 80% of cases; blood, protein and casts are present in the urine and should be examined by dipstick testing and microscopy. If untreated, there is loss of renal function, often within days. Other features include purpuric rashes, nail fold infarcts, and ocular manifestations including conjunctival haemorrhages, scleritis, uveitis, keratitis, proptosis or ocular muscle paralysis due to retro-orbital inflammation. The disease can affect the gut, causing haemorrhage; the heart, causing coronary artery ischaemia; and the neurological system, causing sensory neuropathy or mononeuritis multiplex. The two pathological hallmarks of Wegener's disease are chronic granulomatous inflammation and vasculitis. Granulomas in the lung may coalesce into large masses which cavitate, mimicking tumours (Figure 10.5).

Box 10.2 **Definitions of medium sized vessel vasculitis**

Polyarteritis nodosa
- Necrotizing inflammation of medium and small arteries without glomerulonephritis, pulmonary capillaritis or disease of other arterioles, capillaries or venules

Kawasaki disease
- Arteritis affecting large, medium and small arteries and associated with mucocutaneous lymph node syndrome
- Coronary arteries are usually affected and aorta and veins may be affected
- Usually occurs in children

Box 10.3 **Features of mucocutaneous lymph node syndrome in Kawasaki disease**

- Fever for >5 days
- Conjunctival congestion
- Changes to lips and oral cavity: dry, red, fissured lips; strawberry tongue; reddening of oral and pharyngeal mucosa
- Changes of peripheral extremities: red palms and soles; indurative oedema; desquamation of finger tips during convalescence
- Macular polymorphous rash on trunk
- Swollen cervical lymph nodes

At least five features must be present

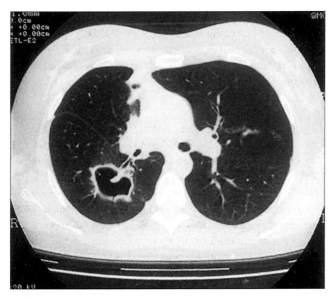

Figure 10.5 Cavitating granulomatous lesion in right lung of patient with Wegener's granulomatosis

Microscopic polyangiitis (microscopic polyarteritis)

Microscopic polyangiitis has many similarities to Wegener's granulomatosis, but disease of the upper respiratory tract is uncommon in microscopic polyangiitis, although pulmonary haemorrhage may occur. Patients with microscopic polyangiitis usually have glomerulonephritis, and, rarely, disease may be limited to the kidney. No granuloma formation is seen.

Diagnosis

Diagnosis is based on typical clinical features, tissue biopsy and the presence of ANCAs (Box 10.4). Sometimes ANCA tests are negative, particularly if disease is limited to the upper respiratory tract (Table 10.1). Antibody titres usually fall, and may disappear completely when the disease is in remission.

Treatment

Treatment of Wegener's granulomatosis and microscopic polyangiitis comprises induction of remission and then maintenance of remission. The intensity of immunosuppression should be determined by the severity of the disease (Box 10.5). For moderate and severe disease, induction treatment should comprise cyclophosphamide and prednisolone, with the addition of methylprednisolone or plasma exchange for patients with severe disease. Patients with mild disease may respond to methotrexate with prednisolone, although response rates are less good. Relapses occur in 40–50% of patients during the first 5 years, so lifelong monitoring for recurring disease activity is essential.

Churg–Strauss syndrome

Churg–Strauss syndrome is associated with an atopic tendency, usually asthma. It may affect coronary, pulmonary, cerebral and splanchnic circulations. Rashes with purpura, urticaria and subcutaneous nodules are common. Glomerulonephritis may develop, but renal failure is uncommon. Diagnosis depends on the presence of typical clinical features, biopsy of skin, lung and kidney, and blood eosinophilia. About 25% of patients are positive for cytoplasmic ANCAs (cANCAs), 50% for perinuclear ANCAs (pANCAs) and 25% have no ANCAs. Patients without poor prognostic features may respond adequately to corticosteroids alone; those patients with poor prognostic features require additional immuosuppression usually with cyclophosphamide. The optimal length of immunosuppression for Churg–Strauss syndrome has not been established, and relapse rates remain high. Asthma requires conventional treatment, but the recently introduced leukotriene receptor antagonist drugs have been causally linked with Churg–Strauss syndrome and should be avoided in these patients.

Box 10.4 Definitions for diagnosis of vasculitides often associated with antineutrophil cytoplasmic antibodies

Wegener's granulomatosis
- Granulomatous inflammation of the respiratory tract
- Necrotizing vasculitis affecting small to medium sized vessels (capillaries, venules, arterioles and arteries)
- Necrotizing glomerulonephritis is common

Microscopic polyangiitis (microscopic polyarteritis)
- Necrotizing vasculitis with few or no immune deposits affecting small vessels (capillaries, venules, arterioles and arteries)
- Necrotizing arteritis of small and medium sized arteries may be present
- Necrotizing glomerulonephritis is very common
- Pulmonary capillaritis often occurs

Churg–Strauss syndrome
- Eosinophil-rich and granulomatous inflammation of respiratory tract
- Necrotizing vasculitis affecting small to medium sized vessels
- Blood eosinophilia (>1.5 × 10⁹/l)
- Usually associated with asthma

Table 10.1 Specificity and sensitivity of ANCA serology testing for Wegener's granulomatosis and microscopic polyangiitis

	Specificity/ sensitivity (%)
Specificity of assays (related to disease controls)	
Indirect immunofluorescence:	
cANCA	95
pANCA	81
ELISAs	
PR3-ANCA	87
MPO-ANCA	91
Combined indirect immunofluorescence and ELISA:	
cANCA/PR3-ANCA positive	99
pANCA/MPO-ANCA positive	99
Sensitivity of combined testing	
Wegener's granulomatosis	73
Microscopic polyangiitis	67

Adapted from Hagen et al., 1998.

Small vessel vasculitis without antineutrophil cytoplasmic antibodies

Henoch–Schönlein purpura

Henoch–Schönlein purpura (Box 10.6) is mainly a disease of children and is usually self-limiting, requiring nothing more than supportive care. The typical features comprise purpura over the buttocks and lower limbs (Figure 10.6), haematuria, abdominal pain, bloody diarrhoea and arthralgia. The pathological hallmarks are deposition of immunoglobulin A (IgA) at the dermoepidermal junction and within the glomerular mesangium, with a mesangial hypercellular glomerulonephritis. Some patients develop a glomerular lesion resembling that seen in small vessel vasculitis. The renal disease may occur in isolation without any other typical manifestations.

Bowel involvement can cause severe bleeding and intussusception, and renal involvement with the development of nephritis can result in renal failure. Prednisolone early in the course of the disease may reduce the abdominal pain and time to resolution of symptoms, and may also reduce the risk of long-term renal disease in patients with Henoch–Schönlein purpura.

Cryoglobulinaemic vasculitis ('mixed, essential')

Cryoglobulins are immunoglobulins that precipitate in the cold. The mixed cryoglobulin consists of a monoclonal IgM rheumatoid factor complexed to polyclonal IgG. Vasculitis (Box 10.6) develops when cryoglobulins deposit in blood vessels. Mixed essential cryoglobulinaemia is due to hepatitis C virus (HCV) infection in >80% of cases. Other causes of cryoglobulinaemia include dysproteinaemias, autoimmune diseases and chronic infections. Serum complement C4 and C3 concentrations are reduced. Clinical features include palpable purpura, arthralgia, distal necroses, peripheral neuropathy, abdominal pain and glomerulonephritis (Figure 10.7).

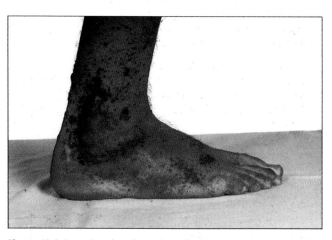

Figure 10.6 Purpuric rash on lower limb of patient with Henoch–Schönlein purpura

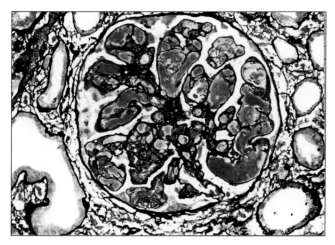

Figure 10.7 Renal biopsy specimen showing intraglomerular deposit of cryoglobulins

The evidence base for treatment of cryoglobulinaemia with or without HCV is still limited. The majority of case series in the literature support the use of a combination of interferons with or without ribavarin to suppress HCV replication, and some form of immunosuppression.

Steroids and cyclophosphamide have been widely used to suppress antibody formation and inflammation in acute disease, although this may be poorly tolerated and lead to increased viral load. Plasma exchange is widely used to remove circulating autoantibodies. There are also case series reporting the use of the anti-B-cell antibody rituximab to reduce the circulating cryoglobulins and control disease.

Isolated cutaneous leukocytoclastic vasculitis

This condition (Box 10.6) is often associated with a drug hypersensitivity response and improves when the drug is stopped. Occasional patients may require corticosteroids for severe disease.

Antiglomerular basement membrane antibody-mediated disease (Goodpasture's disease)

No CHCC definition exists for this rare disease. The hallmarks are a rapidly progressive global and diffuse glomerulonephritis, as seen in small vessel vasculitides, or the presence of pulmonary haemorrhage, or both. Diagnosis depends on finding antibodies to glomerular basement membrane in the serum and linear staining for IgG along the glomerular basement membrane. The antibodies, which are directed against the α3-chain of type IV collagen, have been implicated in disease pathogenesis. About 15–30% of patients have detectable ANCAs. Treatment is with cyclophosphamide and steroids with the addition of plasma exchange to remove circulating antibodies. There is a low probability of recovery of renal function once patients are dialysis dependent, and treatment may be less intensive for this group of patients if there is no evidence of lung involvement.

Further reading

Ballinger S. Henoch–Schönlein purpura. *Curr Opin Rheumatol* 2003;**15**:591–594.

Braun GS, Horster S, Wagner KS *et al.* Cryoglobulinaemic vasculitis: classification and clinical and therapeutic aspects. *Postgrad Med J* 2007;**83**:87–94.

Hagen EC, Daha MR, Hermans J *et al.* Diagnostic value of standardized assays for anti-neutrophil cytoplasmic antibodies in idiopathic systemic vasculitis. EC/BCR Project for ANCA Assay Standardization. *Kidney Int* 1998;**53**:743–753.

Jennette JC, Falk RJ, Andrassy K *et al.* Nomenclature of systemic vasculitides. Proposal of an international consensus conference. *Arthritis Rheum* 1994;**37**:187–192.

Morgan MD, Harper L, Williams JM *et al.* Anti-neutrophil cytoplasm antibody associated glomerulonephritis. *J Am Soc Nephrol* 2006;**17**:1224–1234.

Sunderkötter C, Sindrilaru A. Clinical classification of vasculitis. *Eur J Dermatol* 2006;**16**:114–124.

Weyand CM, Goronzy JJ. Medium- and large-vessel vasculitis. *N Engl J Med* 2003;**349**:160–169.

CHAPTER 11

Varicose Veins

Ali Arshad, Nick JM London, Mark McCarthy

OVERVIEW

- Truncal varicose veins affect 40% of men and 32% of women. Over 80% of people have reticular varices or telangiectasia.
- Trunk varices can cause itching, heaviness, tension or aching.
- Approximately 30% of patients presenting with varicose veins require reassurance and an explanation that their symptoms are not related to their varicosities.
- Surgery has been shown to improve the quality of life in patients with symptomatic varicose veins.
- The place of newer treatments is not yet clear. It is likely that all of the currently available treatments have a role to play. The precise role of these treatments or a combination of treatments remains to be defined.

Introduction

Varicose veins are tortuous, dilated or elongated superficial veins. Size alone, unless the enlargement is gross, does not indicate abnormality, because the size of veins may vary, depending on ambient temperature and hormonal factors in women. In addition, normal superficial veins in a thin individual may appear large, whereas varicose veins in an obese individual may be hidden. Varicose veins can be classified as trunk, reticular or telangiectasia (Figure 11.1). Telangiectasia are also referred to as spider veins, star bursts, thread veins or matted veins. The majority of varicose veins are primary, with only the minority being secondary to conditions such as DVT, pelvic tumours or arteriovenous fistulae.

Incidence and prevalence

The Edinburgh vein study, of people aged 18–64 years, found that truncal varicose veins affected 40% of men and 32% of women. Over 80% of the same population had reticular varices or telangiectasia. There are few studies on the incidence of varicose veins; however, the Framingham study found that the 2-year incidence of varicose veins was 39.4/1000 for men and 51.9/1000 for women.

ABC of Arterial & Venous Disease, 2nd edn. Edited by R. Donnelly and N. London.
© 2009 Blackwell Publishing Ltd. 9781405178891.

Pathophysiology and risk factors

The traditional concept that varicose veins result from failure of valves in the superficial veins leading to venous reflux and vein dilatation has been superseded by the hypothesis that valve incompetence follows rather than precedes a change in the vein wall. Thus, the vein wall is inherently weak in varicose veins, which leads to dilatation and separation of valve cusps so that they become incompetent. This latter theory is strongly supported by the observation that the dilatation of varicose veins is initially distal to the valve, whereas, if the primary abnormality was descending valve incompetence, the initial dilatation should be proximal to the valve.

Risk factors for varicose veins include increasing age and parity, and with occupations that require a lot of standing. There is no evidence that social class, smoking or heredity influence the prevalence of varicose veins. It has been noted that obesity is associated with the development of varicose veins in women, but not in men.

Symptoms

There is often no clear correlation between the appearance of varicosities and the onset of symptoms experienced by the patient. Patients frequently ascribe a myriad of symptoms to their varicose veins. It is important to clarify for patients which of their symptoms are caused by their varicose veins so that they understand which symptoms might improve with treatment. The Edinburgh Vein Study compared the prevalence of symptoms in men and women with and without varicose veins. In men, the only symptom that was significantly associated with trunk varices was itching, whereas, in women, heaviness or tension, aching and itching were significantly associated with trunk varices. No association was found between reticular varices and lower limb symptoms in either men or women (Box 11.1).

Box 11.1 **Symptoms of varicose veins**

- Aching
- Heaviness
- Itching
- Tension

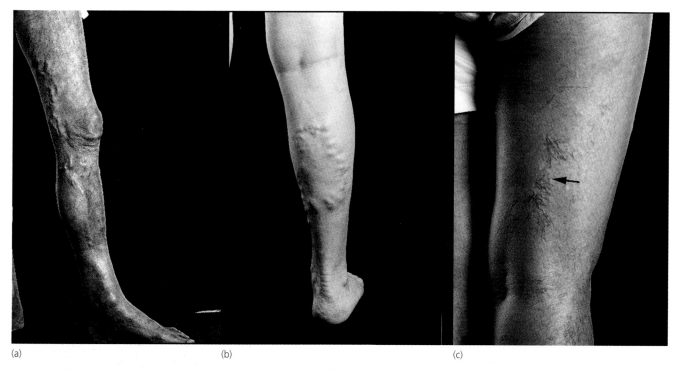

(a)   (b)   (c)

Figure 11.1 Trunk varices are varicosities in the line of the long (a) or short (b) saphenous vein or their major branches. Reticular veins (c) are dilated tortuous subcutaneous veins not belonging to the main branches of the long or short saphenous vein, and telangiectasia (c) are intradermal venules <1 mm in size. c demonstrates both reticular veins (arrow) and telangiectasia. The latter are also referred to as 'spider veins', 'star bursts', 'thread veins' or 'matted veins'

Complications (Box 11.2)

Some complications of varicose veins, such as haemorrhage and thrombophlebitis (Figure 11.2), result from the varicose veins themselves, whereas others, such as oedema, skin pigmentation (Figure 11.3), varicose eczema (Figure 11.4), atrophie blanche (Figure 11.5), lipodermatosclerosis (Figure 11.6) and venous ulceration (Figure 11. 7) result from venous hypertension. There appears to be little relationship between the size of varicose veins and the degree of venous hypertension. Indeed, 40% of limbs with ulceration due to superficial venous incompetence do not have visible varicose veins. Venous ulceration is discussed in Chapter 15.

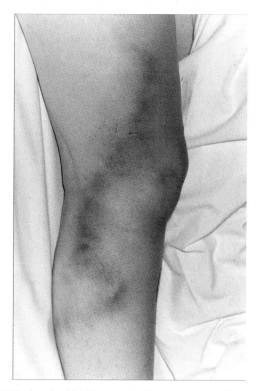

Figure 11.2 Thrombophlebitis presents with severe pain, erythema, and pigmentation over and hardening of the vein. Thrombophlebitis in varicose veins results from stasis, whereas thrombophlebitis occurring in normal veins should alert the clinician to the possibility of an underlying malignancy or thrombophilia. Recurrent thrombophlebitis in varicose veins should also alert the clinician to the possibility of an underlying thrombophilia

Box 11.2 **Complications of varicose veins**

- Bleeding
- Thrombophlebitits
- Oedema
- Skin pigmentation
- Atrophie blanche
- Varicose eczema
- Lipodermatosclerosis
- Ulceration

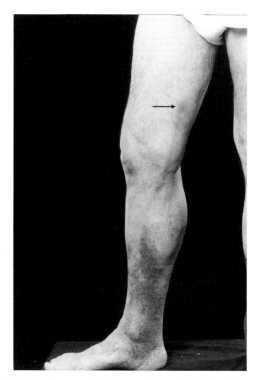

Figure 11.3 Skin pigmentation is due to haemosiderin deposition and is most commonly situated above the medial malleolus. However, it may encircle the entire ankle and extend up the leg. In addition, this patient has thrombophlebitis of the long saphenous vein with overlying pigmentation (arrow)

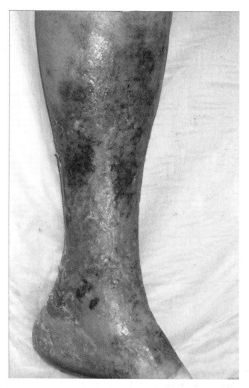

Figure 11.4 Varicose eczema occurs over prominent varicose veins and in the lower third of the leg. It may be dry, scaly and vesicular, or 'weeping and ulcerated'. A generalized sensitization may occur, leading to patches elsewhere. Varicose eczema can be exacerbated by medicaments and dressings, many of which can themselves cause a contact dermatitis

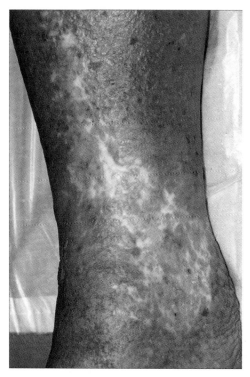

Figure 11.5 Atrophie blanche results from skin necrosis followed by scarring. Sometimes small areas of atrophie blanche coalesce to form a large scar

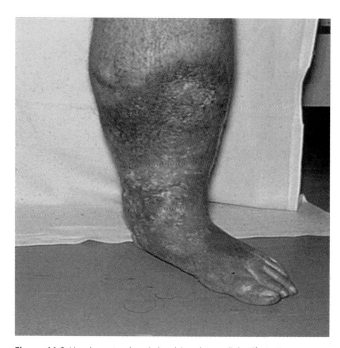

Figure 11.6 Lipodermatosclerosis involving the medial calf. Acute lipodermatosclerosis presents with a painful, tender, hot, raised red-brown area on the lower leg. The chronic form leads to a hard, indurated area on the lower leg with a palpable edge. The overlying skin is often brown and shiny. The progressive contraction of the gaiter area gives the leg an 'inverted champagne bottle' appearance

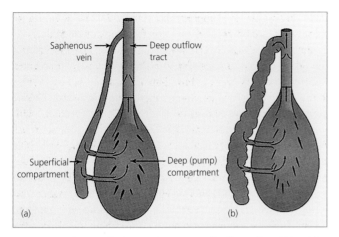

Figure 11.7 The superficial veins do not normally allow reflux of blood (a). However, if the superficial veins are incompetent (b), a proportion of the blood ejected by the calf muscle pump during systole refluxes back down the superficial veins into the calf muscle pump during diastole. This 'retrograde circuit' can volume overload the calf muscle pump, leading to calf muscle pump dilatation and failure. The subsequent rise in end-diastolic volume leads to venous hypertension

Patient assessment

History

It is important to determine precisely why the patient has sought treatment. Thus, it has been found that one-third of patients presenting with varicose veins have symptoms unrelated to their varicose veins or have fears of deterioration or the development of complications. Such patients simply need reassurance. It should be recorded whether the patient has had any episodes of DVT or thrombophlebitis and whether there is a strong family history of DVT. This is important because a history of DVT or thrombophlebitis increases the risk of DVT after varicose vein surgery and may lead to a decision not to operate at all. Patients with a history of DVT or thrombophlebitis who do undergo surgery should receive peri-operative subcutaneous heparin prophylaxis. It is important to note whether females are on the contraceptive pill or taking hormone replacement therapy (HRT). It should also be noted whether there is a history of skin changes because these patients are at an increased risk of developing ulceration.

Examination and investigation

An abdominal examination should be performed to detect any masses which could be causing secondary varicose veins. The patient should be examined standing up. The distribution of the varicosities should be noted, in particular whether they appear to be affecting the long or short saphenous systems, or both. Skin changes and ulceration should be noted. Hand-held continuous-wave Doppler is a simple, readily available tool which can reliably identify the site of incompetence in most primary varicosities. However, its reliability is diminished in recurrent varicose veins and in identifying multiple sites of incompetence and it cannot assess the deep venous system. Most vascular units now employ colour duplex ultrasound scanning to identify sites of superficial incompetence comprehensively and to assess the deep venous system.

Venous duplex scanning is mandatory in any patient with skin changes, ulceration, recurrent varicose veins or with a history of DVT or thrombophlebitis.

Treatment

Approximately 30% of patients presenting with varicose veins require reassurance that their symptoms are not related to their varicosities, or do not have any symptoms and, therefore, do not require any treatment. Reticular varices are not connected to major trunk varices and therefore the treatment options are sclerotherapy or avulsion through small stab incisions. Patients who present with capillary telangiectasia only should undergo colour duplex scanning because ~25% will have clinically unapparent long or short saphenous incompetence. Treatment of the telangiectasia themselves is by microinjections, laser or high-intensity light. If treatment of truncal varicosities is indicated, it can be conservative with compression hosiery or interventional.

Compression hosiery

Patients with aching or oedema as their main symptoms may benefit from compression hosiery. This should be either class I or class II hosiery. If it is uncertain whether the patient's symptoms are caused by varicose veins, a trial of compression hosiery may help: a response to compression indicates that surgery may be beneficial.

Traditional surgery

Surgery has been shown to improve the quality of life in patients with symptomatic varicose veins and reduces the rate of ulcer recurrence in patients with varicose ulceration and normal deep veins. Surgery is directed at treating the cause of the incompetence. Saphenofemoral junction incompetence can be treated by ligation of the junction, stripping of the long saphenous vein in the thigh and multiple avulsions of varicosities. The majority of patients can be treated as a day-case. Most can drive a week later and return to work between 1 and 3 weeks later depending on their occupation. Whilst the incidence of major complications such as bleeding caused by arterial injury or DVT is <1%, about 17% of patients will suffer minor complications. These include temporary saphenous or sural neuralgia caused by damage to sensory nerves when the affected vein is stripped. The rate of recurrent varicose veins after surgery is 20–30% at 10 years.

New interventions

Although injection sclerotherapy has been used for many years, its popularity had waned recently because of concerns about skin staining (Figure 11.8) and a reccurence rate of up to 65% at 5 years. A recent advance has been the introduction of foam sclerotherapy. This involves mixing the sclerosant with a small amount of air or carbon dioxide to produce a foam. The foam pushes the blood throughout the veins and causes vein spasm. Duplex ultrasonography is used to monitor the spread of sclerosant throughout the veins. Complications include skin hyperpigmentation, necrosis, allergic reactions, transient scotoma and confusional states. DVT has also been reported. The treated leg is compressed for up to 2 weeks after treatment. The initial 3-year results are promising.

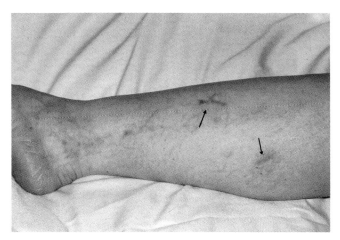

Figure 11.8 One of the complications of injection sclerotherapy is brown skin pigmentation (arrows)

crepe bandaging to compress the vein and thereby minimize thrombus propagation, analgesia—preferably a non-steroidal anti-inflammatory drug (NSAID)—and low-dose aspirin. Patients should be referred to a vascular specialist and consideration given to curative surgery because thrombophlebitis tends to be recurrent if the underlying venous abnormality is not corrected. Colour duplex studies have shown that up to 25% of patients with superficial thrombophlebitis have underlying DVT, and it has therefore been suggested that all patients with thrombophlebitis should undergo duplex scanning to exclude DVT. However, this approach is not practical, and a more realistic suggestion is that patients with phlebitis extending up the long saphenous vein towards the saphenofemoral junction should undergo urgent duplex scanning. If on duplex, thrombus extends into the femoral vein then consideration should be given to urgent saphenofemoral ligation (Box 11.3).

Endovenous laser therapy (EVLT) (Figure 11.9) and radiofrequency ablation (RFA) involve cannulation of the distal long or short saphenous vein under local anaesthesia and the passage of a catheter proximally. Either laser energy or a high-frequency alternating current is delivered, which causes heating of the blood and subsequent vein ablation. In effect, these techniques are alternatives to stripping the long saphenous vein, and either phlebectomies or sclerotherapy are frequently required to remove residual varicosities. Complications include skin burns and DVT. Current safety and efficacy data do support the use of EVLT and RFA, but long-term results are lacking.

Management of complications

Thrombophlebitits

There is no indication for antibiotics in patients with thrombophlebitis. The management of thrombophlebitis includes

> Box 11.3 **Management of thrombophlebitis**
>
> • Crepe bandaging to compress vein and minimize propagation of thrombus
> • Analgesia (preferably a non-steroidal anti-inflammatory drug)
> • Low-dose aspirin

Bleeding

This is dealt with in the acute situation by elevation of the foot above the level of the heart and the application of compression. The patients should then be seen by a vascular surgeon with a view to correcting the underlying abnormality if possible. If the patient has deep venous incompetence that cannot be corrected, then compression hosiery should be worn.

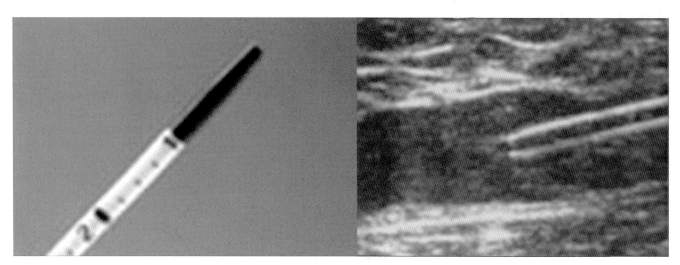

Figure 11.9 Endovenous laser therapy catheter tip. The duplex image shows the catheter within the long saphenous vein

Skin changes and venous ulceration

Patients with haemosiderin staining, varicose eczema or lipodermatosclerosis should undergo colour duplex scanning to define the underlying venous abnormality. Generally, if the only abnormality is superficial venous incompetence then this should be corrected. If, however, the deep veins are incompetent, then superficial surgery will not help and the mainstay of treatment is a topical steroid followed by compression hosiery.

Varicose veins, DVT, the contraceptive pill and HRT

Whilst varicose veins increase the risk of DVT following major abdominal or orthopaedic surgery, there is no evidence that primary varicose veins are a risk factor for spontaneous DVT. Similarly, there is no evidence that women with varicose veins who take the oral contraceptive pill or HRT are at increased risk of DVT compared with women without varicose veins. There is evidence, however, that women with varicose veins who take the pill are more likely to develop thrombophlebitis, and therefore a history of thrombophlebitis is a contraindication to starting the pill and an indication for stopping the pill in current takers. Although not evidence based, the same considerations should probably apply to HRT.

Further reading

Bradbury AW, Evans CJ, Allap PL *et al.* What are the symptoms of varicose veins? Edinburgh vein study cross sectional population survey. *BMJ* 1999;**318**:353–356.

Campbell B. Varicose veins and their management. *BMJ* 2006;**333**:287–292.

Jia X, Mowatt G, Burr JM *et al.* Systematic review of foam sclerotherapy for varicose veins. *Br J Surg* 2007;**94**:925–936.

Mundy L, Merlin TL, Fitridge RA *et al.* Systematic review of endovenous laser treatment for varicose veins. *Br J Surg* 2005;**92**:1189–1194.

Subramonia S, Lees TA. The treatment of varicose veins. *Ann R Coll Surg Engl* 2007;**89**:96–100.

van Rij AM. Varicose veins. *Br J Surg* 2006;**93**:131–132.

CHAPTER 12

Venous Thromboembolic Disease

Akhtar Nasim, Nick JM London

OVERVIEW

- Venous thromboembolism is a common problem in hospitalized patients.
- Diagnosis of deep-vein thrombosis can be established by use of D-dimer testing and compression ultrasonography.
- Pulmonary embolism is a serious and often fatal complication of venous thromboembolism.
- Pulmonary embolism can be diagnosed by spiral CT.
- All at-risk patients must receive thromboprophylaxis.

Introduction

Venous thromboembolism (VTE) is the formation of a thrombus in a vein which may dislodge from its site of origin and travel to another site in the body (embolism). The thrombus forms most commonly in the deep veins of the legs (deep-vein thrombosis; DVT). The dislodged thrombus may travel to the lungs resulting in pulmonary embolism (PE) which can be fatal. In the absence of thromboprophylaxis, the incidence of VTE ranges from 10–20% in general medical patients to 80% in trauma patients, spinal injury patients and patients in the intensive care unit. Therefore, all hospitalized patients should be assessed for the risk of VTE and administered appropriate thromboprophylaxis.

Deep-vein thrombosis

Classically DVT presents with swelling, pain and discoloration of the affected extremity (Figure 12.1). The majority of DVTs arise in the soleal veins of the calf. Thrombosis results from venous stasis or slow flowing blood around venous valve sinuses. Propagation of the clot leads to deep venous obstruction and risk of thromboembolism if the clot dislodges. Examination may reveal a swollen calf, warmth and dilated superficial veins. Box 12.1 lists the differential diagnoses that should be considered in a patient with a painful

swollen leg. Physical examination findings are often unreliable and cannot be used to exclude the diagnosis of DVT. The risk factors for DVT are listed in Table 12.1. DVT of the lower extremity is subdivided into either distal (calf veins) or proximal (thigh) vein thrombosis. Proximal DVT poses the greatest risk of PE and merits anticoagulant therapy.

Diagnosis of DVT

The clinical diagnosis of DVT is very unreliable. Homan's sign described in old text books is of no value. There is no single ideal investigation for diagnosing DVT. A D-dimer test has a high negative predictive value and can therefore be used to rule out DVT (if not elevated). It enables near-patient testing and can therefore be used in a general practice setting. The finding of an elevated D-dimer concentration alone is insufficient to establish the diagnosis of DVT, as elevated levels are not specific for VTE and are commonly present in those with malignancy, recent surgery, trauma or pregnancy. A venogram is the gold standard investigation for establishing the diagnosis of DVT (Figure 12.2). However, it is invasive, involves use of contrast (can cause allergic reactions and nephrotoxicity) and the procedure is sometimes technically difficult. It has now largely been replaced by compression ultrasonography (Figure 12.3). Compression ultrasonography is considered to be the best non-invasive diagnostic method and has a sensitivity and specificity of ~97% for proximal DVT. A clinical model has been developed

---

Box 12.1 **Differential diagnosis of DVT**

- Calf muscle injury
- Acute lipodermatosclerosis
- Superficial thrombophlebitis
- Lymphatic insufficiency/lymphoedema
- Ruptured Baker's cyst
- Leg swelling in a paralysed limb
- Cellulitis
- Knee joint pathology
- Fracture
- Reperfusion injury/compartment syndrome

ABC of Arterial & Venous Disease, 2nd edn. Edited by R. Donnelly and N. London.
© 2009 Blackwell Publishing Ltd. 9781405178891.

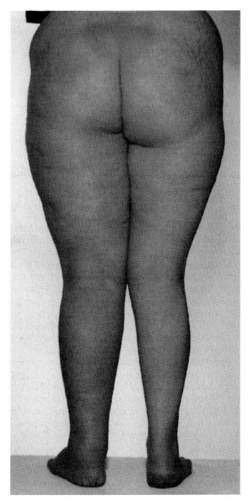

Figure 12.1 Photograph of a patient with a swollen left leg due to iliofemoral venous thrombosis

Table 12.1 Risk factors for venous thromboembolism

Acquired disorders	Inherited/congenital disorders
Malignancy	Antithrombin deficiency
Surgery, especially orthopaedic	Protein C deficiency
Presence of central venous catheter	Protein S deficiency
Trauma	Factor V Leiden mutation
Pregnancy, HRT, oral contraceptive	Prothrombin gene mutation
Prolonged immobilization	Dysfibrinogenaemias
Congestive cardiac/respiratory failure	Factor VII/XII deficiency
Antiphospholipid syndrome	
Myeloproliferative disorders	
Poorly controlled diabetes mellitus	
Hyperviscosity syndromes (e.g. myeloma)	
Inflammatory bowel disease	
Acute medical illness	
Age > 60 years	
Behcet's disease	
Obesity (BMI > 30)	
Varicose veins associated with phlebitis	

BMI = body mass index; HRT = hormone replacement therapy.

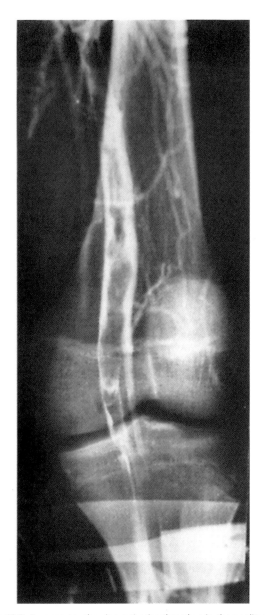

Figure 12.2 A venogram showing extensive thrombus in the popliteal vein

which takes into account symptoms, signs and risk factors and can be applied to categorize patients as having a low or high probability of DVT (Table 12.2). This has been demonstrated to be reproducible and has been used to develop an algorithm incorporating D-dimer testing and compression ultrasonography which simplifies the management of patients suspected of having DVT (Figure 12.4). Other non-invasive investigative modalities which offer potential for simplifying the diagnosis of VTE include spiral CT and MRI.

Complications of DVT

The main complications of DVT are PE, post-thrombotic venous insufficiency and recurrence of thrombosis.

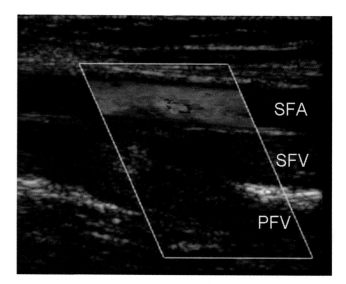

Figure 12.3 A compression ultrasound image demonstrating normal flow in the superficial femoral artery (SFA) with no flow in the superficial femoral vein (SFV) and profunda femoris vein (PFV) both of which contain echogenic thrombus

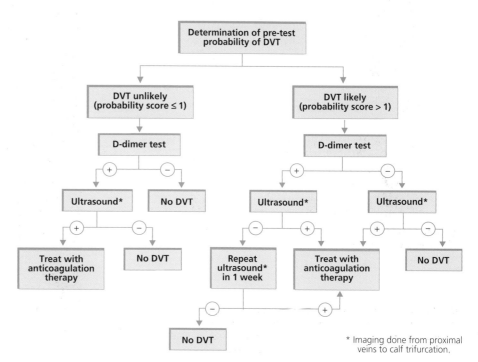

Figure 12.4 Algorithm for diagnosis of deep-vein thrombosis (reproduced from Scarvelis and Wells, 2006)

* Imaging done from proximal veins to calf trifurcation.

Table 12.2 Clinical model for predicting pre-test probability of deep-vein thrombosis (Wells' score)

Clinical characteristic	Score
Active malignancy (treatment ongoing or within 6 months or palliative)	1
Paralysis, paresis or recent plaster immobilization of lower limbs	1
Recently bedridden for >3 days or major surgery within previous 12 weeks	1
Localized tenderness along the distribution of the deep venous system	1
Whole leg swollen	1
Calf swelling >3 cm compared with the normal leg (measured 10 cm below tibial tuberosity)	1
Pitting oedema (only affecting the symptomatic leg)	1
Collateral superficial veins (non-varicose)	1
Previously documented DVT	1
Alternative diagnosis at least as likely as DVT	−2

DVT likely, score ≥ 2; DVT unlikely, score ≤1.
Low probability of DVT, ≤0; high probability of DVT, score ≥3.
Modified from Scarvelis and Wells (2006).

Box 12.2 **Clinical features of pulmonary embolism**

- Dyspnoea/tachypnoea
- Pleuritic chest pain
- Cough
- Haemoptysis
- Pyrexia
- Tachycardia
- Central cyanosis
- Elevated jugular venous pressure
- Accentuated pulmonary component of second heart sound
- Circulatory collapse

Pulmonary embolism

PE is a serious complication and is associated with 1–8% mortality despite adequate therapy. A massive PE results from a large embolus that obstructs the main pulmonary artery, leads to acute right ventricular failure and is generally fatal. Smaller emboli lodge more distally in the pulmonary arterial tree and are more likely to produce pleuritic chest pain. Most PEs are multiple and affect the lower lobes in the majority of the cases. The most common symptoms are dyspnoea, pleuritic pain, cough and haemoptysis (see Box 12.2), although some patients with PE have no symptoms at the time of the diagnosis. The gold standard for diagnosing PE is a pulmonary angiogram. However, this has now largely been replaced by spiral CT (Figure 12.5). The latter is non-invasive, widely available and can detect other lung disease if there is no PE. A ventilation/perfusion scan (V/Q scan) may be a useful alternative in patients who have contrast allergy or in pregnancy due to a lower radiation exposure than CT. The majority of patients with PE are treated with anticoagulation and supportive measures. Massive PE resulting in haemodynamic instability (hypoxia, tachycardia and hypotension) is an indication for thrombolysis. Surgical management of massive acute PE has been largely abandoned due to poor outcomes.

Post-thrombotic venous insufficiency

DVT can lead to venous valve damage, resulting in valvular incompetence. A combination of deep-vein reflux and venous obstruction from unresolved thrombus leads to post-thrombotic venous insufficiency (also known as post-phlebitic syndrome). The cumulative incidence of this condition is 17, 23 and 28% at 1, 2 and 5 years, respectively, with no increase thereafter. It results in lower leg swelling, pain, skin pigmentation and venous ulcers (Figure 12.6). The trophic skin changes (haemosiderin deposition, lipodermatosclerosis, atrophie blanche, skin ulceration) tend to occur 2–4 years after DVT. The use of class II compression hosiery in patients with DVT has been shown to reduce the incidence of this complication.

Recurrent thrombosis

The recurrence of DVT is associated with a high risk of further thromboembolic events. Therefore, such patients should probably continue with life-long anticoagulation.

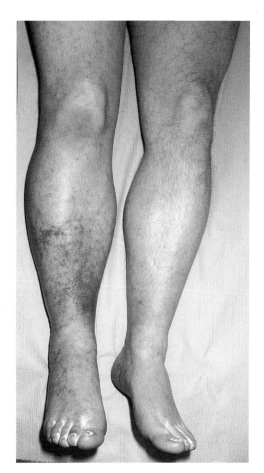

Figure 12.6 A photograph showing the typical skin changes observed in patients with post-thrombotic venous insufficiency (right leg)

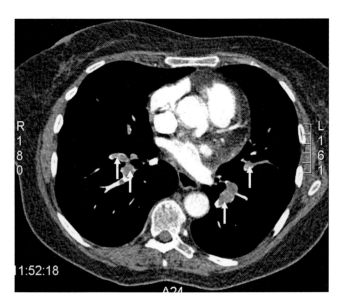

Figure 12.5 A spiral CT image showing bilateral thrombi (arrows) within the major branches of the pulmonary arteries

Treatment of deep-vein thrombosis

Anticoagulation

A patient with a proximal vein thrombosis (involving the deep thigh veins) requires anticoagulation. This prevents the propagation of thrombus and PE in the short term and prevents recurrent events in the long term (see Chapter 17).

Inferior vena cava filter

These can be used physically to prevent embolization of the thrombi and hence reduce the rate of PE. They are indicated in patients who cannot be safely anticoagulated (recent haemorrhage and impending surgery) or patients who continue to develop PE despite adequate anticoagulation (see Chapter 17).

Elastic compression stockings

Below-knee elastic compression hosiery (class II) reduces venous stasis in the lower leg by applying a graded degree of compression to the ankle and calf, with greater pressure being applied distally. They reduce the oedema and prevent blistering which can occur as a result of the venous hypertension. Use of elastic compression stockings following a DVT reduces the risk of developing post-thrombotic venous insufficiency.

Prevention of venous thromboembolic disease

All patients should be assessed on admission to identify their risk for developing VTE. Patients undergoing surgery should be fitted with graduated compression/antiembolism stockings unless contraindicated (patients with arterial insufficiency or diabetic neuropathy). In addition to the above mechanical prophylaxis, patients at increased risk of VTE (one or more risk factors—see Table 12.1)

should be commenced on low molecular weight heparin (LMWH). Fondaparinux may be used as an alternative to LMWH as it is associated with a substantially lower risk of heparin-induced thrombocytopenia (HIT). The NICE recommendation is that patients undergoing major orthopaedic surgery should continue with LMWH or Fondaparinux for 4 weeks after surgery. Patients should continue to use compression/antiembolism stockings until their level of mobility returns to normal. Vena caval filters should be considered for those patients with recent (within 1 month) or current VTE in whom anticoagulation is contraindicated (see above). The thromboprophylaxis regime should be reviewed on daily ward rounds to ensure that there is compliance with the recommended guidelines.

Acknowledgements

We would like to thank Dr J Enwistle, Consultant Radiologist, for providing Figure 12.5 and Mr T Hartshorne for Figure 12.3.

Further reading

Greer I, Hunt BJ. Low molecular weight heparin in pregnancy: current issues. *Br J Haematol* 2005;**128**:593–601.

National Institute for Health and Clinical Excellence. *Venous thromboembolism: reducing the risk of venous thromboembolism (deep-vein thrombosis and pulmonary embolism) in inpatients undergoing surgery*. (NICE) clinical guideline 46. April 2007.

Scarvelis D, Wells PS. Diagnosis and treatment of deep-vein thrombosis. *CMAJ* 2006;**175**:1087.

Wells PS, Owen C, Doucette S *et al*. Does this patient have deep-vein thrombosis? *JAMA* 2006;**295**:199–207.

White RH. The epidemiology of venous thromboembolism. *Circulation* 2003;**107**(Suppl 1):14–18.

CHAPTER 13

Lymphoedema

Vaughan Keeley

OVERVIEW

- Lymphoedema is more common than was once thought.
- Although the condition is incurable, patients can usually be helped by a combination of physical treatments.
- There is no effective drug treatment.
- Cellulitis is an important complication which should be treated promptly with antibiotics.

Introduction

Lymphoedema is a swelling of the tissues as a result of a failure of lymphatic drainage. When it first develops the swelling is mainly due to the accumulation of fluid, but over time fibrosis and adipose tissue is deposited.

In the past, lymphoedema has been considered to be uncommon and untreatable. This situation has changed in recent years, and this chapter describes the current position.

Lymphoedema/chronic oedema

All oedema arises from an imbalance of capillary filtration and lymphatic drainage (Box 13.1). Therefore, technically, all oedema has a lymphatic component. For example, in venous disease, capillary filtration is increased as a result of increased venous pressure. This leads to an increase in lymphatic drainage to match it. When the transport capacity of the lymphatic system is exceeded, capillary filtration exceeds lymphatic drainage and oedema develops (high output failure of the lymphatics in a venous oedema). However, over time, the increased flow in the lymphatics declines, probably as a result of vessel damage, and a further failure of lymphatic drainage develops (lymphoedema).

In immobile patients, a chronic 'dependency' oedema of the legs commonly develops ('armchair legs'). This arises from a failure of the muscle pump in the legs to propel both blood and lymph in the veins and lymph vessels, respectively. Thus venous pressure and therefore capillary filtration is increased and lymphatic flow is reduced, resulting in a lymphovenous oedema.

In pure lymphoedema lymphatic failure is of two types:

1. *Primary lymphoedema*. This is due to an abnormality of development of the lymphatic system.
2. *Secondary lymphoedema*. This arises from an extrinsic process which damages a normal lymphatic system, e.g. surgery, trauma, radiotherapy and infection (cellulitis, filariasis).

In clinical practice, pure lymphoedema may be relatively uncommon, but many patients have chronic oedema which may have a lymphatic component. These patients suffer similar problems to those with pure lymphoedema. Thus the umbrella term 'chronic oedema' is useful both clinically to describe the range of conditions and in epidemiological studies looking at its prevalence and aetiology.

Prevalence of chronic oedema

'Chronic oedema' has been defined as an oedema of >3 months duration affecting any part of the body: limbs and mid-line structures, e.g. head and neck, trunk and genitalia. In a study carried out in a population in SW London, the prevalence was found to be 1.33 per 1000 population overall. This makes it as common as venous leg ulcers. Prevalence increased with age, rising to 5.4 per 1000 in those aged >65 years and 10.3 per 1000 in those >85 years.

The prevalence of the different types of oedema is not clear from the literature. Even in cancer treatment-related oedema, there is a wide range of incidences reported (Box 13.2). This is partly as a result of the difficulty in defining what constitutes a significant oedema. For example, in studies of arm oedema developing after the treatment of breast cancer, lymphoedema may be defined as a percentage excess in limb volume of the affected limb compared with the unaffected limb, e.g. >5% or >10%, or a change in limb volume or circumference post-surgery compared with that pre-operatively, e.g. >100 or >200 ml difference. Thus, depending upon the definition used, incidence may vary between studies. In addition, the length of follow-up affects the measured incidence as lymphoedema can develop many years after treatment, particularly radiotherapy. Finally, newer treatment techniques, e.g. sentinel node biopsy, should result in a reduced frequency of lymphoedema so older published figures may be higher than more recent ones.

ABC of Arterial & Venous Disease, 2nd edn. Edited by R. Donnelly and N. London.
© 2009 Blackwell Publishing Ltd. 9781405178891.

Box 13.1 **Factors causing lymphoedema/chronic oedema**

Factors causing an increased capillary filtration
- Increased venous pressure, e.g. in venous disease, deep-vein thrombosis, heart failure, immobility
- Increased capillary pressure due to arteriolar dilation, e.g. angioedema, and drugs, e.g. nifedipine
- Reduced plasma oncotic pressure, e.g. in hypoalbuminaemia

Factors causing reduced lymphatic drainage
- Structural damage to lymphatic vessels, e.g. due to surgery and/ or radiotherapy
- Developmental abnormality in lymphatic vessels, e.g. hypoplasia in Milroy's disease.
- Reduced 'muscle pump' activity in immobility

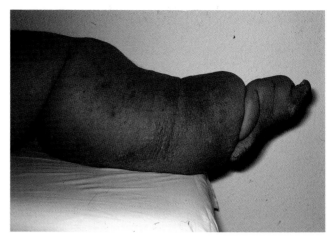

Figure 13.1 Lymphoedema of the leg showing shape distortion and increased skin creases

Box 13.2 **Incidence of lymphoedema following cancer treatments**

- Breast cancer: 1–54%
- Gynaecological cancers: 1–70%
- Genitourinary cancers: 10–100%
- Malignant melanoma of the leg: 6–80%

Box 13.3 **Changes in skin and subcutaneous tissues in established lymphoedema**

- Thickened, dry skin
- Hyperkeratosis (build up of horny layer)
- Lymph blisters (dilated lymphatics, lymphangiectasia)
- Papillomatosis (dilated lymphatics with fibrosis causing a cobblestone appearance)
- Increased skin creases around joints, e.g. ankles
- Chronic inflammatory skin changes
- Positive Stemmer's sign (inability to pick up a fold of skin over the proximal phalanx of the second toe, reflecting swelling and thickening of subcutaneous tissues)

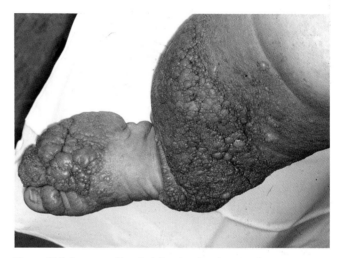

Figure 13.2 Severe papillomatosis in a lymphoedematous leg

Box 13.4 **Symptoms of lymphoedema**

- Swelling of limb or other area
- Pain: ache, heaviness or tightness of limb
- Pain: shoulder or hip/back pain due to mechanical effect of weight of limb
- Reduced mobility/use of limb
- Stiffness of joints
- Leakage of fluid (lymphorrhoea)
- Body image/psychological issues (inability to wear desired clothing/shoes; difficulty getting items to fit; difficulty with appearance of limb)

Nevertheless, the general theme is that the more damage done to the lymphatic system during treatment, the more likely it is for the patient to develop lymphoedema.

Clinical features of chronic oedemas

The features of chronic oedemas depend upon their aetiology. Chronic venous disease is described elsewhere (Chapter 15). This chapter will focus on the specific features of lymphoedema.

When lymphoedema first develops it appears as a soft, pitting swelling which does not have any specific features. However, with time, as a result of a chronic inflammatory process, fibrosis and adipose tissue accumulate in the subcutaneous tissues causing the swelling to become firmer and less easy to 'pit'. At the same time, typical skin changes develop (Box 13.3; Figures 13.1 and 13.2).

Patients with lymphoedema also experience a number of symptoms (Box 13.4). The impact of chronic lymphoedema on a patient's quality of life is often underestimated by healthcare professionals. It can present a significant physical, psychological, social and financial burden.

Complications of lymphoedema

The most important complications are shown in Box 13.5.

Cellulitis represents a major clinical problem for people with lymphoedema. The susceptibility to cellulitis and the development of new malignancies is believed to be due to a local immune deficiency as a result of an impairment of the normal role of the lymphatic system in the immune response.

DVT, especially of the legs, may occur in individuals with lymphoedema, due to immobility.

Lymphorrhoea is the leakage of lymph through the skin through either injury to the skin or rupture of lymphangiectasia or papillomata.

Diagnosis of lymphoedema and other chronic oedemas

Lymphoedema is usually diagnosed on the basis of the history and examination. A family history may be present in those with primary lymphoedema, and a cause should be evident in those with secondary lymphoedema, e.g. treatment for breast cancer. The clinical features described above should be sought.

Other important causes of chronic oedema are included in Box 13.6, although this list is not exhaustive. These should be considered in the differential diagnosis.

Lipoedema

Lipoedema is a type of lipodystrophy in which there is an abnormal deposition of fat in the legs and lower part of the body, usually in women. This presents as a non-pitting enlargement of the legs usually noticed from puberty onwards. Supra-added pitting oedema can develop, particularly in the feet and ankles (known as lipolymphoedema).

Investigations

In the early stages of lymphoedema the diagnosis may not be straightforward as the appearances of the swelling, skin and subcutaneous tissues may be non-specific, and investigations, e.g. lymphoscintigraphy and ultrasound, may be helpful.

Lymphoscintigraphy

This involves the subcutaneous injection into a webspace in the foot or the hand (depending on the area being investigated) of a radiolabelled macromolecule (e.g. 99mTc nanocolloid) which is absorbed into the lymphatics from the interstitial space. The passage of the tracer is followed using a gamma camera and sequential images are taken, ideally until the tracer reaches the root of the limb and beyond.

Lymphoscintigraphy of the leg will be considered further here as this is the most commonly performed.

In a normal lymphoscintigram, the tracer flows up the leg through a small number of lymphatics to reach the inguinal nodes within 30–45 min. In lymphoedema, the appearance of the tracer in the inguinal nodes is delayed and the tracer may take alternative routes (collaterals) in the skin ('dermal backflow') and the deep (subfascial) lymphatic system such that an outline of the skin and the popliteal nodes are demonstrated (Figure 13.3). Other abnormal patterns of flow can also be seen.

Ultrasound examination

Ultrasound examination of the veins and soft tissues of the legs may be helpful in distinguishing venous oedema and other causes of swelling such as lipoedema.

Treatment of lymphoedema

The main treatment for lymphoedema (and some other chronic oedemas) is a combination of physical therapies (Box 13.7).

There is evidence that the combination of treatments is effective in reducing both limb volume and the incidence of cellulitis, but the contribution of each component and whether all elements are needed in all patients is not clear. In response to this lack of a firm evidence base, an international consensus document on the management of lymphoedema has been published recently.

Patients may require two phases of treatment:

1. An intensive phase of on average ~2 weeks duration in which compression bandaging is applied and renewed often on a daily basis. Manual lymphatic drainage (MLD) may be employed as part of this phase.
2. A maintenance phase comprising the wearing of a compression garment and skin care, with the application of a moisturizer,

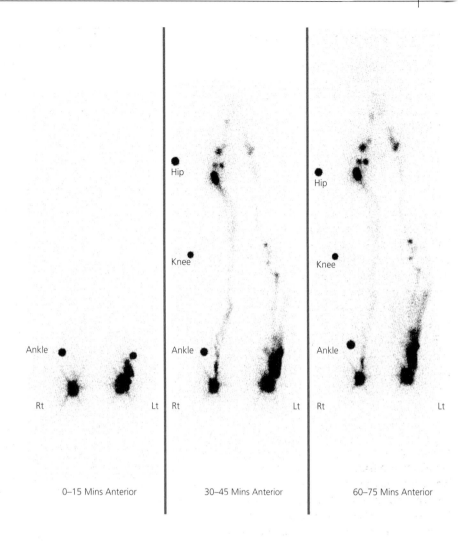

Hip

Knee

Ankle

Rt   Lt

Hip

Knee

Ankle

Rt   Lt

Hip

Knee

Ankle

Rt   Lt

0–15 Mins Anterior   30–45 Mins Anterior   60–75 Mins Anterior

Figure 13.3 Lymphoscintigram showing lymphoedema of the left leg with delayed flow of tracer to inguinal nodes, the visualization of popliteal nodes and dermal backflow

---

Box 13.7 **Physical treatments of lymphoedema**

Compression:
- Multilayer lymphoedema bandaging using short stretch bandages
- Elastic compression garments

Massage:
- Manual lymphatic drainage (MLD): a light massage technique applied by trained professionals designed to improve lymphatic drainage
- Simple lymph drainage (SLD): a modification of MLD which can be carried out by the patient or carer

Exercise:
- Exercise whilst wearing compression garments increases lymph drainage

Skin care:
- Use of moisturizers to improve the hydration of dry skin
- Prompt treatment of athlete's foot
- Treatment of skin conditions, e.g. eczema
- Taking precautions to minimize trauma, e.g. wearing gloves when gardening, avoiding walking with bare feet

both on a daily basis. Simple lymphatic drainage (SLD) may form part of this phase.

Some patients with mild oedema may be managed with the 'maintenance phase' approach only.

The contraindications to compression treatment are shown in Box 13.8.

The combination of physical treatments requires significant patient concordance to be successful and, in those with oedema associated with other chronic illnesses, help is usually required for skin care, putting on and taking off compression garments, etc.

Box 13.8 **Some contraindications/cautions in compression treatment**

- Acute DVT (concerns about encouraging embolism)
- Acute cellulitis (painful)
- Peripheral vascular disease (concerns about causing worse ischaemia)
- Acute heart failure (concerns regarding exacerbating failure)

Box 13.9 Summary of oral treatment for cellulitis in lymphoedema

- Amoxicillin 500 mg 8 hourly for at least 14 days
- Flucloxacillin 500 mg 6 hourly should be added if evidence of Staphylococcal infection, e.g. folliculitis, crusted eczema
- If allergic to penicillin, clindamycin 300 mg 6 hourly instead of the above

Drug therapies

Diuretics

Pure lymphoedema does not respond to loop diuretic therapy. However, in chronic oedema of a more complex aetiology involving fluid retention or an element of heart failure, diuretics may have a place.

Benzopyrones

A number of benzopyrones, e.g. coumarin and oxerutins, have been investigated to determine their role in the management of lymphoedema. There is some evidence of a beneficial effect, but a recent Cochrane Review concluded that this was insufficient to support their routine use. Coumarin has been withdrawn due to hepatotoxicity.

Management of cellulitis in lymphoedema

Cellulitis typically presents with 'flu-like symptoms followed by the appearance of a painful, red, hot swelling of the lymphoedematous area. It is believed to be mainly due to infection with β-haemolytic Streptococci, although many patients are treated with anti-Staphylococcal antibiotics. The evidence base for the best treatment of cellulitis is limited. Consensus guidelines have been developed recently (see Box 13.9 for summary).

Patients may often be managed with oral antibiotics at home, but some, with severe systemic upset, may require i.v. antibiotics and bed rest in hospital.

Patients with lymphoedema may experience recurrent episodes of cellulitis.

If this occurs, the management of the swelling should be reviewed, as it is known that a reduction in limb volume is associated with a reduction in the incidence of cellulitis. Sources of infection, e.g. ingrowing toenails, eczema and athlete's foot, should be treated appropriately. In those experiencing two or more episodes per year, prophylactic antibiotics are recommended: phenoxymethylpenicillin 500 mg per day or erythromycin 500 mg per day if the patient is allergic to penicillin.

Conclusions

Lymphoedema/chronic oedemas are more common than previously thought. Although incurable, they can usually be helped by a combination of physical treatments and the appropriate management of complications, particularly cellulitis.

Further reading

Badger C, Preston N, Seers K, Mortimer P. Benzopyrones for reducing and controlling lymphoedema of the limbs. *Cochrane Database Syst Rev* 2003;(4):CD003143.

BLS/LSN. Consensus guidelines on the management of cellulitis in lymphoedema available at www.thebls.com and www.lymphoedema.org/lsn. 2007

Keeley VL. The role of lymphoscintigraphy in the management of chronic oedema. *J Lymphoedema* 2006;**1**:42–57.

Lymphoedema Framework. *Best practice for the management of lymphoedema. International consensus.* London: MEP Ltd, 2006.

Moffatt CJ, Franks PJ, Doherty DC *et al.* Lymphoedema: an underestimated health problem. *Q J Med* 2003;**96**:731–738.

Williams AF, Franks PJ, Moffatt CJ. Lymphoedema: estimating the size of the problem. *Palliat Med* 2005;**19**:300–313.

CHAPTER 14

The Ulcerated Lower Limb

Nick JM London, Richard Donnelly

OVERVIEW

- Ulceration of the lower limb affects 1% of the total adult population and 3.6% of the population over the age of 65 years.

- Venous hypertension, arterial impairment and neuropathy account for >90% of all lower limb ulcers.

- Leg ulcers are painful and markedly reduce quality of life. Painless leg ulceration can occur in patients with a severe sensory neuropathy. Diabetes is the most common cause of neuropathy in the UK.

- It is important to examine lower limb sensation carefully. This is best done with a monofilament.

- The mainstay of leg ulcer treatment is to establish the aetiology and then treat the underlying pathology. Wound dressings do not produce healing but rather provide the optimum environment for healing once the underlying pathology has been corrected.

Box 14.1 **Aetiology of leg ulcers**

- Venous hypertension
- Arterial impairment
- Neuropathy
- Mixed venous–arterial
- Trauma
- Obesity or immobility
- Vasculitis
- Calciphylaxis
- Malignancy
- Underlying osteomyelitis
- Pressure ulcers
- Blood dyscrasias
- Necrobiosis lipoidica diabeticorum
- Pyoderma gangrenosum
- Infection
- Lymphoedema

Introduction

Ulceration of the lower limb affects 1% of the total adult population and 3.6% of the population over the age of 65 years. Leg ulcers are debilitating and painful, and it has been shown that patients with leg ulcers have a markedly reduced quality of life that is restored by ulcer healing. Lower limb ulceration tends to be recurrent, and it has been estimated that the total annual cost of leg ulceration to the UK National Health Service is £600 million.

Aetiology (Box 14.1)

Venous hypertension, arterial impairment and neuropathy account for >90% of all lower limb ulcers. It is useful to divide leg ulcers into those occurring in the gaiter area and those occurring in the forefoot. This is because the aetiologies in these two sites are different (Figure 14.1). It has been reported that at least two aetiological factors can be identified in one-third of all lower limb ulcers.

ABC of Arterial & Venous Disease, 2nd edn. Edited by R. Donnelly and N. London.
© 2009 Blackwell Publishing Ltd. 9781405178891.

Venous ulcers result from venous hypertension and most commonly occur above the medial or lateral malleoli (Figures 14.2 and 14.3). Venous hypertension may result from venous disease or from calf muscle pump failure. The most common causes of calf muscle pump failure are obesity and arthritis of the hip, knee or ankle. Arterial ulcers frequently involve the toes, shin or occur over pressure points (Figure 14.4). Atherosclerosis is by far the most common underlying arterial pathology.

Neuropathic ulcers tend to occur on the sole of the foot or over pressure points (Figure 14.5). The most common cause of neuropathic ulcers is diabetcs. Other causes of neuropathy include alcohol abuse, drugs and vitamin B deficiency. Diabetic patients at high risk are those with worsening peripheral sensory neuropathy, poor diabetes control, delayed presentation to carers and high alcohol consumption. It is important to note that apart from necrobiosis lipoidica, diabetes is not a primary cause of ulceration but leads to ulceration through neuropathy or ischaemia, or both.

Painless mechanical trauma is the most common reason for ulceration developing in the feet of diabetic patients. Poorly fitting shoes precipitate build up of callus over areas of high pressure and it is typically in these areas that ulcer formation follows. Foot

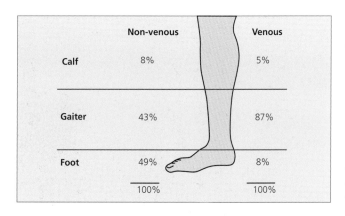

	Non-venous	Venous
Calf	8%	5%
Gaiter	43%	87%
Foot	49%	8%
	100%	100%

Figure 14.1 The causes of ulceration in the calf, gaiter area and forefoot. The majority of venous ulcers occur in the gaiter area. The majority of non-venous ulcers are due to arterial disease and/or neuropathy and occur in the foot

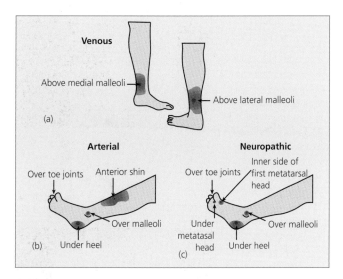

Figure 14.2 The common sites of venous (a), arterial (b) and neuropathic (c) ulceration.

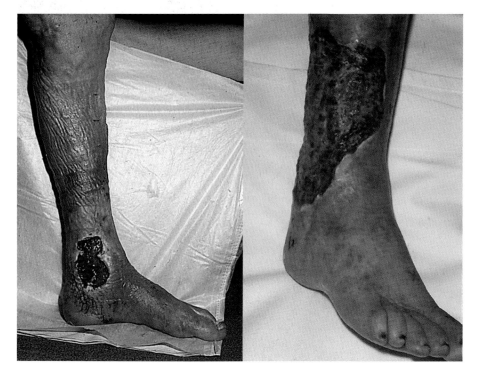

Figure 14.3 The most common sites for venous ulceration are above the medial or lateral malleolus

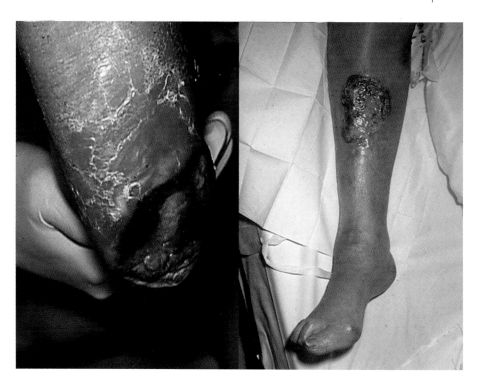

Figure 14.4 Arterial ulcers can affect the shin or pressure points such as the heel

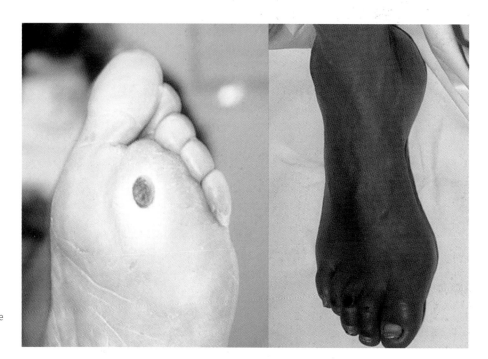

Figure 14.5 Neuropathic ulcers occur on the sole of the foot and over the dorsum of the toe joints. The foot with ulceration of the dorsum of the toe joints has associated infection and lymphangitis

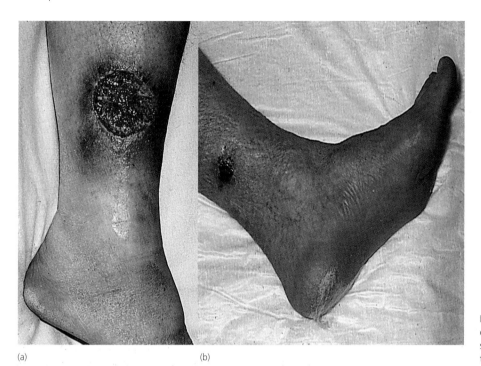

(a)   (b)

Figure 14.6 Malignancy, such as squamous cell carcinoma (a) or basal cell carcinoma (b), should be borne in mind in leg ulcers that fail to heal despite adequate treatment

deformities are very common in diabetic patients and develop for a variety of reasons. Patients with a motor neuropathy develop claw-toes, and the dorsal surface of these clawed-toes may rub within their shoes and lead to ulceration. A proportion of patients develop a progressive and destructive deforming arthropathy. This deformity is known as Charcot's foot or arthropathy, and leads to areas of high pressure on the diabetic foot which then leads to ulceration.

The possibility of malignancy (Figure 14.6), particularly in ulcers that fail to start healing after adequate treatment, should always be borne in mind. The most common malignancies are basal cell carcinoma, squamous cell carcinoma and melanoma. The most common causes of vasculitic ulcers are rheumatoid arthritis, systemic lupus erythematosus and polyarteritis nodosa. The blood dyscrasias that most commonly lead to leg ulceration are sickle cell disease, thalassaemia, thrombocythaemia and polycythaemia rubra vera. Venous disease affects up to 30% of the population and it is therefore not uncommon for patients with, for example, rheumatoid arthritis or a blood dyscrasia to have venous disease causing their lower limb ulceration. Thus, in up to half of patients with rheumatoid arthritis and leg ulcers, the ulceration is due to venous disease rather than to the rheumatoid arthritis.

Lymphoedema rarely ulcerates spontaneously, but ulceration can occur secondary to trauma or immobility. Calciphylaxis occurs in patients undergoing haemodialysis, patients with hyperparathyroidism or idiopathically, and leads to skin ulceration through intravascular calcification and thrombosis. The most common conditions associated with pyoderma gangrenosum (Figure 14.7) are inflammatory bowel disease, rheumatoid arthritis and lymphoproliferative disorders. Although infective causes of leg ulceration are rare in the UK, infections such as tuberculosis, syphilis, yaws, leprosy and cutaneous leishmaniasis are common in many parts of the world. Indeed, leishmaniasis is the most common cause of skin ulceration worldwide.

Clinical assessment

History

It is important to enquire about the duration of ulceration and whether it is a first episode or recurrent. Whilst recent trauma can precipitate arterial, venous or neuropathic ulceration, a history of severe past trauma raises the possibility of underlying osteomyelitis. Pain is a major problem for patients with leg ulcers. Patients

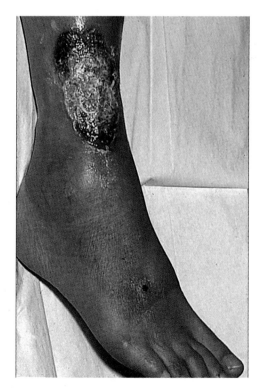

Figure 14.7 Pyoderma gangrenosum. This patient has Crohn's disease

Table 14.1 Ulcer edge characteristics

Edges	Ulcer type
Sloping	Venous ulcer
Punched out	Arterial or neuropathic
Rolled	Basal cell carcinoma
Everted	Squamous cell carcinoma
Undermined	Pressure or tuberculosis
Purple	Pyoderma gangenosum

with chronic sensory neuropathy often complain of paraesthesia and sharp, stabbing, shooting or burning pain which is worse at night. The absence of pain may indicate severe sensory neuropathy. A history of claudication or rest pain (pain in the foot at night relieved by dangling the foot out of bed) indicates underlying arterial disease. A history of varicose veins, DVT or immobility raises the possibility of underlying venous hypertension. A history of systemic diseases that may be associated with leg ulceration should be noted. These diseases include blood dyscrasias, rheumatoid arthritis, inflammatory bowel disease, the vasculitides, renal failure and hyperparathyroidism. Recent travel abroad raises the possibility of an infective cause.

Examination

The ulcer edge should be inspected (Table 14.1) and the surrounding skin should be examined for signs of cellulitis. Cellulitis should not be confused with varicose eczema or lipodermatosclerosis (Table 14.2). Inspection of the leg should include a search for signs of venous hypertension. These are haemosiderin pigmentation, varicose eczema, atrophie blanche and lipodermatosclerosis. The presence of varicose veins should be noted. In diabetic patients, autonomic neuropathy may lead to the foot becoming dry, cracked and fissured. The ulcers of pyoderma gangrenosum have a violaceous overhanging edge. Vasculitic ulcers are usually small, multiple, shallow and may be associated with purpura. The peripheral pulse status should be recorded and, in patients with critical ischaemia, Buerger's test will be positive (pallor of the sole of the foot on elevation to 45°).

The patient's gait should be observed, particularly noting whether the calf muscles are employed. Patients with a shuffling or antalgic gait do not use their calf muscle pump and therefore develop venous hypertension. The range of hip, knee and ankle joint move-

ment should be noted. Structural deformities including hammer toes, bunions, calluses and Charcot's arthropathy can lead to pressure ulceration and should be documented.

Sensation should be examined. A tuning fork (128 Hz) is used to assess vibration sense. This should be carried out over the medial malleolus. Pin-prick sensation is often used to assess the protective sensation associated with pain. However, this assessment is prone to interinvestigator variation due to the pressure applied to the pin. A more accurate technique is to use Semmes–Weinstein monofilaments. These monofilaments are placed against the skin and pressure applied until the monofilament buckles. The patient should perceive this sensation and identify the area being touched at the time that the monofilament buckles. A 10 g force (5.07 monofilament) is the upper limit deemed to confer adequate protection from ulceration.

In the case of foot ulceration the patient's shoes must be examined to check that they are not too tight fitting and causing pressure necrosis. Also it is not uncommon to find 'foreign objects' in the shoes of patients with neuropathy. In the case of ulcers involving the sole of the foot, the sole should be carefully examined for signs of ascending infection, including proximal tenderness and the appearance of pus on proximal compression of the sole. Note any surrounding callus, typical of neuropathic ulceration, and look for tracking to involve the bones of the foot. If it is possible to probe to bone there is an 85% probability of underlying osteomyelitis.

Referral

Patients with foot ulceration should be referred to hospital for investigation because many will have underlying arterial ischaemia or neuropathy that requires prompt management. Patients with venous ulceration should have their ABPI measured. If the ABPI is >0.8 these patients can either be managed primarily in the community by trained nurses or may be referred to hospital for investigation into the underlying venous abnormality. Patients with an ABPI <0.8 should be referred to hospital. Patients with ulcers of uncertain aetiology should be referred for hospital investigation. Many of the latter ulcers will require a diagnostic biopsy. In addition, ulcers that look malignant and venous ulcers that fail to heal at all despite adequate compression bandaging should be referred for biopsy. The only indication for swabbing an ulcer is if there is the presence of cellulitis around it.

Table 14.2 Comparison of cellulitis, lipodermatosclerosis and varicose eczema

Cellulitis	Lipodermatosclerosis	Varicose eczema
Red, warm, painful	Red, warm, painful	Red, not warm, not painful
Develops over 24–72 h	Chronic	Chronic
Patient systemically unwell	No systemic symptoms	No systemic symptoms
Fever	No fever	No fever
Well-defined advancing edge	Localized, hard edge	Diffuse
No exudate	No exudate	Exudate
No itch	No itch	Itchy
Not scaly	Not scaly	Scaly
No underlying induration	Underlying induration	No underlying induration

Management

The mainstay of leg ulcer treatment is to establish the aetiology and then correct the underlying problem. Wounds that are covered with slough or eschar need debridement so that healing can occur. Debridement can be sharp using a scalpel, ultrasonically assisted or biological using larval therapy. The wound dressings most commonly used are occlusive and create a moist environment. There are a large number of wound dressings available, and no one dressing has been shown to be superior. The dressing should be as simple as possible. This not only minimizes cost but also reduces the chances of an allergic reaction. It must be stressed that the wound dressing itself does not produce healing, but rather provides the optimum environment for healing once the underlying cause of the ulcer has been addressed. Leg ulceration associated with systemic disease is based primarily on the treatment of the underlying disease. The management of venous ulceration is described in Chapter 15.

Arterial ulceration

In order for arterial ulcers to heal, the underlying arterial abnormality must be corrected. These patients therefore require colour duplex scanning of their arterial system or diagnostic arteriography to define the underlying arterial abnormality. Angioplasty is the treatment of choice (Figure 14.8) because bypass grafting in the presence of ulceration carries an increased risk of wound and/or graft infection. For those patients in whom angioplasty is not possible, some form of bypass operation should be performed, preferably using saphenous vein.

Neuropathic ulceration

Many diabetic patients with neuropathic ulceration will also have an arterial component that requires correction. In many hospitals, diabetic patients with foot ulceration are managed in specialist foot clinics run by a combination of diabetic physicians, vascular surgeons, specialist nurses and podiatrists. The principles behind treatment are to optimize blood supply, to debride callous and dead tissue, to treat active infection, to educate the patient with regard to foot care and to protect the ulcerated area so that healing can occur. In selected patients, MRI of the foot can be invaluable to determine the extent of infection and guide surgical debridement. The wound dressings used should not cause maceration of the surrounding healthy skin, and in the case of plantar ulcers should allow dependent drainage.

There are a number of methods available to reduce plantar pressure, including casts such as the Scotchcast boot and Total-contact boot. The Scotchcast boot is made from fibreglass tape and is lined with felt and soft bandaging that is individually fitted and moulded to the shape of the patient's foot. The boot is removable, allowing regular inspection of the ulcer for debridement and other local

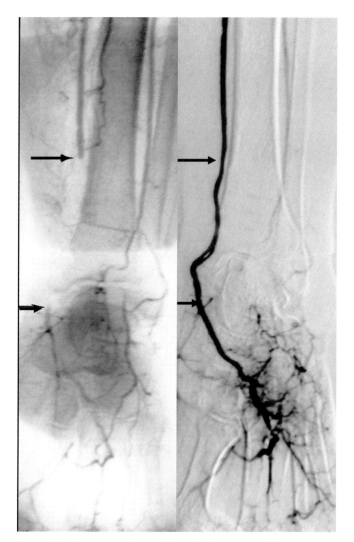

Figure 14.8 An occlusion (arrows) of the distal posterior tibial artery pre- and post-angioplasty . Using modern balloon catheters it is possible to angioplasty stenosed or occluded calf arteries

wound care. Alternatively, a window can be cut out of the boot (Figure 14.9). These lightweight casts allow the patient to remain ambulatory. Plantar ulcers that fail to respond to Scotchcast boots may be encased in a Total-contact cast. This is a close-fitting plaster of Paris and fibreglass cast which holds the foot and lower leg to prevent slipping and rubbing. Most neuropathic plantar ulcers heal within a period of 6–12 weeks within these casts.

Once the cast is removed, the feet should be placed in specialist pressure-relieving footwear to reduce future ulceration and complications developing. This may involve the manufacture of bespoke leather footwear which is made from one piece of material. The shoes should allow plenty of space for the depth and width of the foot, have no internal seams which may precipitate rubbing and should be Velcro-fastened or lace-ups to prevent sliding within the footwear. Additional techniques to reduce abnormally high plantar pressures include specialist insoles contoured to the shape of the sole and rockerbottom soled shoes to alleviate pressure over the metatarsal heads.

Further reading

Cavanagh PR, Lipsky BA, Bradbury AW *et al*. Treatment for diabetic foot ulcers. *Lancet* 2005;**366**:1725–1735.

Grey J, Harding K, eds. *ABC of wound healing*. Oxford, Blackwell BMJ Books, 2006.

Morison M, Moffatt CJ, Franks PJ, eds. *Leg ulcers: a problem-based learning approach*. Mosby Inc., London, 2007.

Negus D, Coleridge-Smith D, Bergan JJ, eds. *Leg ulcers. Diagnosis and management*. Edward Arnold, London, 2006.

Scottish Intercollegiate Guidelines Network. *The care of patients with chronic leg ulcer*. SIGN 26. July 1998.

Scottish Intercollegiate Guidelines Network. *Management of diabetes*. SIGN 55. November 2001.

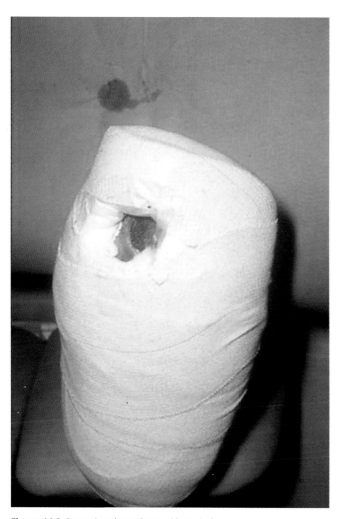

Figure 14.9 Protective plaster boot with a window cut out

CHAPTER 15

Venous Ulceration

Manj S Gohel, Keith R Poskitt

OVERVIEW

- Chronic leg ulceration is a major healthcare expense.
- Venous hypertension is the most commont cause of chronic leg ulceration.
- Patients with leg ulceration require arterial (ABPI) and venous (colour duplex) assessment to plan management.
- Multilayer compression is the most effective therapy to heal venous ulcers.
- The ablation of superficial venous reflux (using surgery, foam sclerotherapy or endovenous ablation) is the best treatment to reduce ulcer recurrence.

Introduction

Venous ulceration is the most common cause of lower limb ulceration in the Western world. Chronic venous hypertension is thought to be the primary cause of ~75% of leg ulcers and may be a significant contributory factor in a further 15% (Figure 15.1). Ulceration represents the end stage of a spectrum of venous disorders affecting the leg and is thought to cost the NHS £400–600 million per year. The prevalence is estimated at 1% in the adult population, but may be as high as 3% in those >65 years of age. This chapter aims to summarize the pathophysiology, assessment and treatment of patients with venous ulceration.

Pathophysiology of venous ulcers

Patients with venous leg ulcers have persistently high pressure in their leg veins. This 'venous hypertension' results from valvular reflux in the venous system due to inherently faulty valves in either deep or superficial venous systems (primary reflux) or following recanalization of a previous DVT where previously competent valves are damaged. Patients who have venous hypertension may have no symptoms or start with small varicose veins, but over time the skin may become inflamed (venous eczema), pigmented (haemosiderinosis) or thickened and scaly (lipodermatosclerosis), and eventually break down, resulting in leg ulceration. The severity of venous disease may be described using the CEAP classification (Table 15.1). The precise mechanism of ulceration following venous hypertension is poorly understood, but the high pressure is thought to push both red and white blood cells and other factors out into the perivascular tissues and cause epithelial cell injury and thus ulceration.

Venous ulcers typically occur in the medial gaiter area of the leg and are commonly seen with other venous skin changes (Figure 15.2). It is important to remember that venous hypertension may also be caused by reduced mobility, obesity, ankle stiffness and poor calf muscle pump function. Moreover, other factors such as malnutrition, co-morbidity and medication may also impair the chance of wound healing. The treatment of patients with venous ulcers should include the correction of these contributing factors where possible, but is primarily aimed at reducing the persistent venous hypertension or its pathophysiological effects.

Assessment

Aims of assessment

Thorough patient assessment is essential to plan an appropriate and individual management plan. The primary aims of assessment are to confirm the aetiology of the ulcer and identify other contributing factors that may delay healing. In addition, the impact of the ulcer on the patient and the expectations from treatment should be considered when choosing a management plan.

History

A detailed history may highlight important aetiological factors and help predict prognosis for individual patients. Symptoms such as varicose veins, skin pigmentation, previous DVT or past episodes

ABC of Arterial & Venous Disease, 2nd edn. Edited by R. Donnelly and N. London.
© 2009 Blackwell Publishing Ltd. 9781405178891.

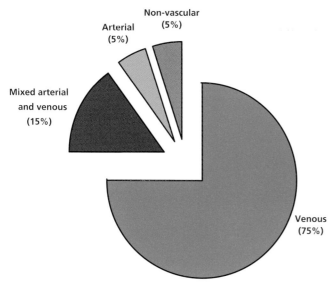

Figure 15.1 The aetiology of chronic leg ulcers

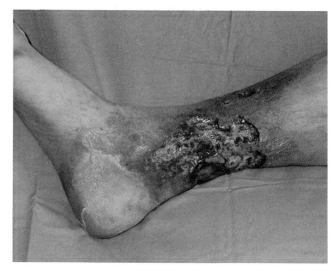

Figure 15.2 A patient with venous ulcer and typical skin changes of venous hypertension

of ulceration may support a venous cause for the leg ulcer. Advanced patient age and ulcer chronicity are independent risk factors for delayed ulcer healing and may be useful to counsel patients of their prognosis. The presence of other pathologies may suggest other diagnoses for the ulceration (e.g. ulcerative colitis and pyoderma gangrenosum). Moreover, the patient's occupation and social circumstances are often important considerations when planning a treatment regimen.

Clinical examination

The examination should include assessment of general health and the ulcerated limb. Poor mobility, malnourishment and other untreated co-existent pathologies may be encountered in the elderly patient group. Examination of the ulcer should include details of the size, shape, margin, ulcer characteristics and precise location. A diagnosis of venous ulceration may be supported by a wound in the medial gaiter area, oedema, skin thickening and pigmentation. However, 20–30% of venous ulcers may occur in other parts of the

lower leg, and skin changes may be present in patients with non-venous causes of ulceration. The use of tracings may allow accurate documentation and objective assessment of the response to treatment.

Investigations
Arterial assessment
Measurement of ABPI is essential in all ulcerated legs to ensure that significant arterial compromise is not present (Figure 15.3). The use of compression is contraindicated in the presence of

Table 15.1 The CEAP classification for venous disorders of the leg

CEAP clinical stage	Description
C0	Absence of any signs of venous disease
C1	Reticular veins
C2	Truncal varicose veins
C3	Oedema
C4	Skin changes (pigmentation, lipodermatosclerosis)
C5	Healed ulceration
C6	Open ulceration

*Other factors included in CEAP are (a)etiological (congenital, primary or secondary), anatomical (superficial, deep or perforator reflux) and pathophysiological (reflux, obstructed or combined).

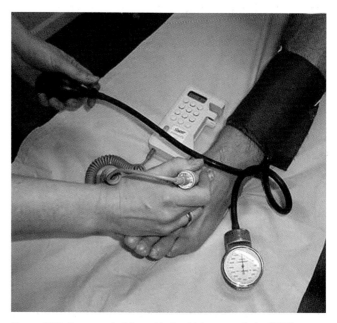

Figure 15.3 Assessment of the ankle–brachial pressure index (ABPI)

severe arterial disease (ABPI <0.5), but patients with moderate arterial compromise (ABPI 0.5–0.80) may be safely treated with modified compression therapy within the setting of a specialist leg ulcer clinic. As arterial disease may progress, patients with non-healing ulcers should have repeat ABPI assessment. It should be noted that falsely elevated ABPIs may be seen, particularly in diabetic patients as a result of calcification within the vessel wall, and also in large legs. Further assessment using toe arterial pressure measurement or colour arterial duplex may be necessary in individual cases.

Venous assessment

Colour venous duplex scanning provides reliable anatomical information about patency and flow direction for superficial and deep veins, and has superseded venography for the assessment of venous disease in the leg. Patients with venous ulceration should undergo duplex assessment in order to identify superficial venous reflux that may be relatively easily treated with surgery, foam injections or other endovenous interventions. While venous duplex scanning provides important anatomical information, it may fail to estimate the severity of venous dysfunction. Other tests of venous function giving more detailed physiological assessment include ambulatory venous pressure monitoring and various plethysmography measurements. Their use is generally limited to research centres and specialist units, but these tests are becoming important tools in patient selection.

Histological assessment

Since 1% of all leg ulcers are malignant, it is recommended that suspicious or non-healing ulcers are biopsied. In our experience, the most common malignancy is basal cell carcinoma (60%) followed by squamous cell carcinoma (40%).

Treatment of venous ulceration

Where should treatment take place?

Patients with venous ulceration have a complex combination of physical, psychological and social morbidities that require a holistic approach to management. In the UK, patients with venous ulcers may be managed in the community by experienced nursing teams, in hospital by vascular surgical services, or a combination of primary and secondary care. The location and model of care provided are usually dependent on local factors, but the care of such patients should ideally include:

- A specialist and enthusiastic clinical team with close links to primary care and hospital resources
- Detailed arterial and venous assessment
- Evidence-based treatment delivered in a convenient friendly clinical setting
- Regular audit of clinical outcomes including 12- and 24-week healing rates and 12-month recurrence rate

A number of studies have evaluated the effectiveness of community-based leg ulcer clinics and protocol-driven patient management. Studies from Charing Cross, Sheffield and Cheltenham have

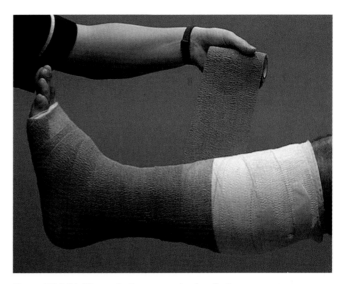

Figure 15.4 Multilayer elastic compression bandaging

demonstrated excellent healing and recurrence rates for patients treated with this model of care.

Treatment to heal the ulcer

The mainstay of treatment for patients with venous ulceration is multilayer graduated compression bandaging applying 40 mmHg of compression at the ankle and 17–20 mmHg to the upper calf (Figure 15.4). The compression therapy reduces the effects of venous hypertension in the ulcerated leg and facilitates wound healing. Healing rates of ~50–60% at 3 months can be achieved using this approach.

Patients are advised to elevate the leg while at rest and to walk regularly to encourage calf muscle pump activity in order to reduce venous hypertension. Smoking cessation should be encouraged and nutritional deficiencies should be addressed. Although the cohort benefits of these conservative measures are unknown, they are considered to be good medical advice. The use of a huge and confusing range of wound dressings has been identified in recent years and treatment regimens have often been devised not by evidence, but by consumerism. Reliable evidence is now available, including a recent meta-analysis which concludes that the type of dressing beneath compression bandages has no effect on ulcer healing. The mainstay of venous ulcer treatment is to correct the underlying pathophysiology by compression, elevation and correction of sustained venous hypertension.

Although numerous systemic medicines have been proposed for venous ulceration, none has been consistently shown to improve wound healing in prospective studies. The use of antibiotics should be reserved for patients with signs of lymphangitis or spreading cellulitis. In patients with excessive slough, wound debridement may be beneficial in order to obtain a healthy granulating bed across which epithelium will spread or skin grafts can flourish. Debridement may occur with compression alone, but can also be

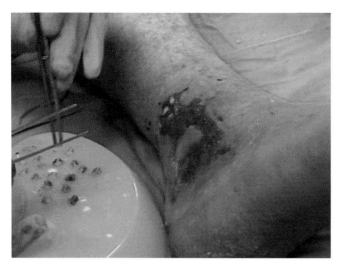

Figure 15.5 Pinch skin grafting may be used to promote ulcer healing in some patients

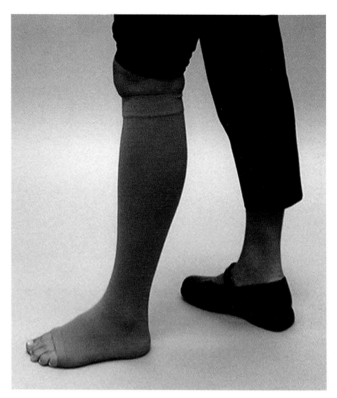

Figure 15.6 Class II elastic stockings can reduce the risk of recurrent ulceration

performed using biological, surgical or larval treatment. Larval therapy (maggots) for wound debridement is generally well tolerated and commonly used.

Skin grafting using either pinch grafts (Figure 15.5) or split skin may be beneficial particularly for larger ulcers in order to encourage epithelial growth. Ulcer excision or shaving to create an 'acute wound' can be performed in combination with skin grafting. In general, additional therapies should be used in combination with compression therapy.

Prevention of recurrence

Without preventative measures, the risk of ulcer recurrence may be as high as 60% within 3 years. While multilayer compression is the mainstay of treatment for venous ulcer healing, ulcer recurrence is minimized by either countering the effects of venous hypertension (e.g. compression stockings) or treating the superficial venous reflux (e.g. surgery, foam or endovenous techniques).

The use of class II elastic compression stockings (providing 18–24 mmHg ankle pressure) reduces the effects of venous hypertension in the leg and lowers the risk of ulcer recurrence (Figure 15.6). Class III stockings (providing 25–35 mmHg ankle pressure) may provide even greater protection against recurrent ulceration, but they are more difficult to wear and patient compliance is poorer. Patients should be advised to wear stockings during the day and may remove them at night. However, this may present a problem to this predominantly elderly population who may suffer with arthritis of the hands or hips and therefore struggle to put on and remove stockings.

Duplex studies have demonstrated that the majority of patients with venous ulceration have reflux affecting the superficial venous system (long or short saphenous veins) which may be treated by standard varicose vein surgery. A recent large randomized trial (ESCHAR trial) demonstrated that surgical treatment of superficial venous reflux can significantly reduce the risk of recurrent leg ulceration. In recent years, numerous minimally invasive endovenous treatment options have gained in popularity and, in some centres, have replaced traditional 'open' varicose vein surgery. New therapies such as foam sclerotherapy (Figure 15.7a–e), laser treatment or radiofrequency ablation may be performed under local anaesthetic and as an outpatient. Early reports of these therapies suggest that venous function in ulcerated legs is improved, and this treatment may be more acceptable to the elderly leg ulcer population than open surgery.

Summary

Venous ulcers are common and expensive to treat. Patient care should be shared between primary and secondary care, and all patients should be entitled to a detailed clinical assessment in a specialist setting to plan an effective management strategy. While multilayer compression therapy is the most effective treatment to heal venous ulcers, continued treatment with compression stockings is considerably less effective than treatment of the refluxing superficial venous system for reducing ulcer recurrence. New endovenous therapies such as foam sclerotherapy may replace surgery for the ablation of superficial venous reflux.

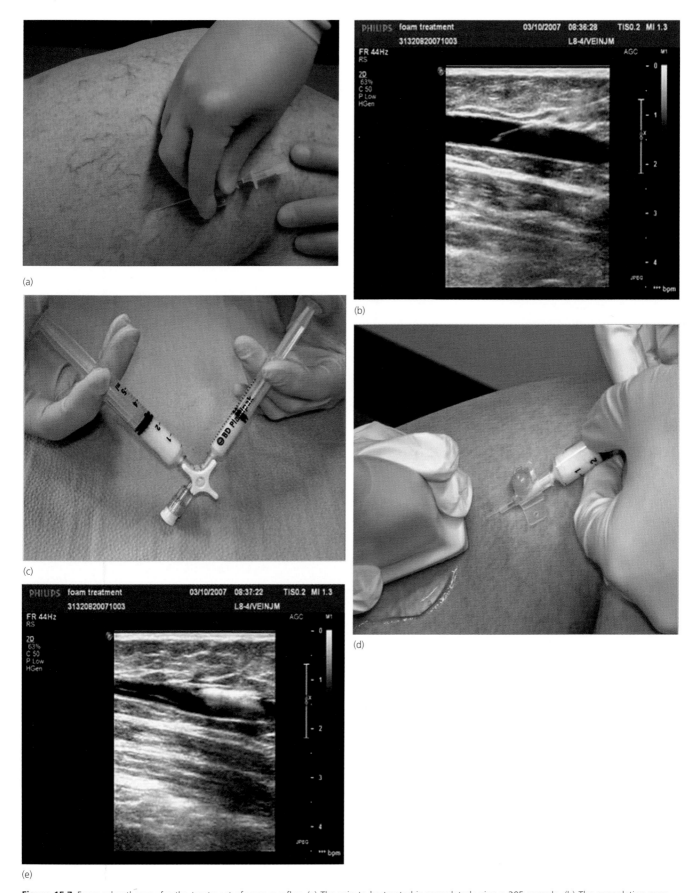

Figure 15.7 Foam sclerotherapy for the treatment of venous reflux. (a) The vein to be treated is cannulated using a 20F cannula. (b) The cannulation may be performed under ultrasound guidance to improve accuracy. (c) Foam is created by mixing sclerosant with air (Tessari technique). (d) The foam is then injected into the vein to be treated. (e) The foam can easily be visualized occluding the vein using duplex ultrasound

Further reading

Adam DJ, Naik J, Hartshorne T *et al*. The diagnosis and management of 689 chronic leg ulcers in a single-visit assessment clinic. *Eur J Vasc Endovasc Surg* 2003;**25**:462–468.

Bergan JJ, Shortell CK. *Venous ulcers*. Academic Press, New York, 2007.

Cullum N, Nelson EA, Fletcher AW *et al*. Compression for venous leg ulcers. *Cochrane Database Syst Rev* 2001;(2):CD000265.

Gohel MS, Barwell JR, Taylor M *et al*. Long term results of compression therapy alone versus compression plus surgery in chronic venous ulceration (ESCHAR): randomized controlled trial. *BMJ* 2007;**335**:83–87.

Ruckley CV, Evans CJ, Allan PL *et al*. Chronic venous insufficiency: clinical and duplex correlations. The Edinburgh Vein Study of venous disorders in the general population. *J Vasc Surg* 2002;**36**:520–525.

CHAPTER 16

Antiplatelet Therapy in Arterial Disease

G Stansby, P Kesteven, DP Mikhailidis

OVERVIEW

- Antiplatelet agents are commonly used in patients with atherosclerosis in order to reduce thrombosis risk.

- The platelet surface membrane is rich in receptors and adhesion proteins that co-ordinate interactions between the platelet, other platelets, components of the blood and the vessel wall, e.g. fibrinogen, vitronectin, von Willebrand factor, collagen, fibronectin and laminin.

- Aspirin acts by irreversibly acetylating cyclooxygenase-1 and -2 (COX-1 and COX-2), thereby inhibiting thromboxane A_2 and vasodilatory prostacyclin (prostaglandin I_2) formation.

- The thienopyridine group of ADP antagonists (clopidogrel and ticlopidine) act on $P2Y_{12}$ receptors.

- Blocking the receptor (glycoprotein IIb/IIIa) responsible for fibrinogen binding is an effective and powerful method of preventing platelet aggregation. Despite their proven use in coronary disease, glycoprotein IIb/IIIa blockers have yet to establish a role in peripheral artery disease particularly with their risks of adverse bleeding. Oral preparations are yet to prove effective.

- NICE has recommended that patients with acute coronary syndromes—who do not undergo percutaneous coronary intervention—should be prescribed clopidogrel and aspirin for 12 months.

- Following ischaemic stroke or transient ischaemic attack, NICE recommend the combination of modified-release dipyridamole and aspirin for 2 years.

Introduction

Platelets are smooth discoid anucleate cells derived from mega-karyocytes which play a central role in haemostasis and in throm-botic disorders. Their average lifespan is usually 7–10 days and normally there are $150–400×10^9$ platelets/l circulating in an inactive state. Donné first identified platelets in 1842, but it was not until 1882 that Bizzozero noted that platelets adhered to vascular lesions and to each other to form 'white thrombi'.

ABC of Arterial & Venous Disease, 2nd edn. Edited by R. Donnelly and N. London. © 2009 Blackwell Publishing Ltd. 9781405178891.

Atheroma produces an inherently thrombogenic inner surface on affected blood vessels. As a result, acute arterial thrombosis can occur, resulting in adverse clinical outcomes such as acute coronary thrombosis. The majority of such events occur where the pre-existing plaque was not causing a critical, flow-limiting, stenosis. The final critical event is thought to be surface plaque rupture with exposure of thrombogenic plaque material. Because of this, anti-platelet agents are commonly used in patients with atherosclerosis in order to reduce thrombosis risk. The groups most commonly considered for antiplatelet agents are those with coronary disease, cerebrovascular disease or peripheral arterial disease (PAD). In itself PAD is often a relatively benign condition with <5% of patients with intermittent claudication (IC) per 5 years deteriorat-ing and requiring peripheral arterial intervention or amputation. The mainstay in managing patients with IC is treating modifiable cardiovascular risk factors to reduce the risk of myocardial infarc-tion and stroke, the main causes of death.

Platelet hyperactivity in atherosclerotic disorders

Patients with various atherosclerotic disorders have highly acti-vated platelets compared with the normal population. This platelet hyperactivity may be the result of a number of factors that are more prevalent in patients with atherosclerosis. Cigarette smoking, hypercholesterolaemia and other established atherosclerotic risk factors are capable of leading directly to platelet activation. In addi-tion, the total surface area of atheroma that platelets are exposed to in the flowing blood is also likely to lead to direct activation of platelets. Although data are conflicting, there may also be a rela-tionship between platelet receptor polymorphisms and propensity to develop arterial disease. Finally, if platelet turnover is increased, relatively 'younger' platelets may be more 'active' than older circu-lating platelets.

Mechanisms of platelet action

Several complex mechanisms are involved in the activation and aggregation of platelets, with final common pathways resulting in amplification of this process (Figure 16.1). The platelet surface membrane is rich in receptors that co-ordinate these interactions

Resting platelets

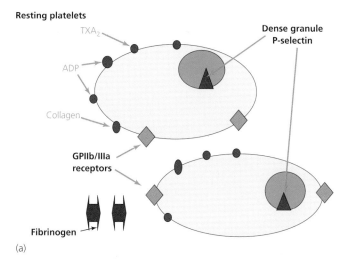

(a)

Activated platelets

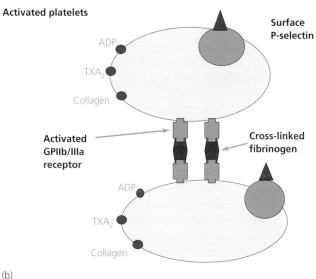

(b)

Figure 16.1 (a) Various agonists such as TXA₂, collagen and ADP can activate platelets by binding to specific receptors. (b) This results in activation of the GPIIb/IIIa receptor and cross-linking by fibrinogen binding, and also fusion of granules with the platelet surface, resulting in surface P-selectin expression

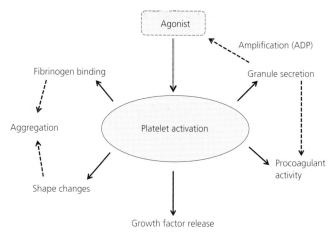

Figure 16.2 Schematic showing how agonist binding results in several processes which include amplification of the initial stimulus resulting in a 'cascade' of activation and recruitment of other platelets

between the platelet, other platelets, components of the blood and the vessel wall. These include surface receptors and adhesion proteins (e.g. fibrinogen, vitronectin, von Willebrand factor, collagen, fibronectin and laminin), many of which are found in the basement membrane of blood vessels, being exposed by disruption of the endothelial layer. Shape change, degranulation and fibrinogen binding are the key processes involved in activation and aggregation of platelets (Figure 16.2).

Important platelet agonists/receptors

ADP/ATP receptors (Figure 16.3)

ADP and ATP are stored in platelet granules and released to reinforce both aggregation and degranulation when platelets are stimulated by a variety of agents. Gaarder first identified ADP as a platelet agonist in 1961, and to date three receptors have been identified. ADP interacts with purinergic P2 surface receptors, divided into the P2Y and P2X subclasses, which are linked with either G-proteins or ion channels, respectively. In response to ADP there is

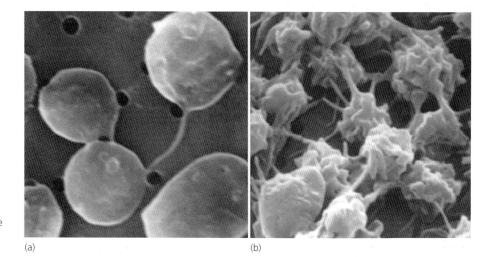

Figure 16.3 Quiescent platelets are shown on the left (a) and activated platelets are shown on the right (b). Activation has resulted in shape change—the platelets have become more rounded and produced pseudopodia

(a)   (b)

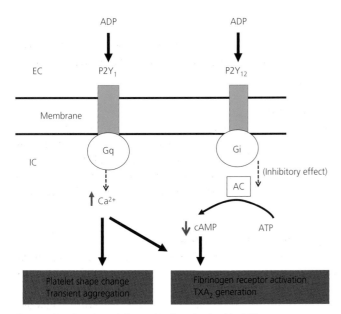

Figure 16.4 Overview of the mechanisms involved in ADP receptor activation. AC = adenyl cyclase; EC = extracellular; Gi = inhibitory G-protein, Gq = excitatory G-protein; IC = intracellular

a rapid rise in cytoplasmic Ca^{2+}, adenyl cyclase inhibition and concomitant activation of G-protein pathways and phospholipase C. The thienopyridine group of ADP antagonists (clopidogrel and ticlopidine) act on $P2Y_{12}$ receptors. Figure 16.4

Collagen receptors
Collagen has a triple-helical structure that is assembled into fibrils, and is an important structural component of connective tissue. Binding of platelets to collagen has an important role in repair of damaged areas of endothelium. Several platelet collagen receptors exist; these receptors are not G-protein linked.

Thromboxane
Receptors for thromboxane A_2 (TXA_2) are found on the surface of platelets and vascular smooth muscle cells. TXA_2 binds to low- and high-affinity binding sites on platelets; the low-affinity site is irreversible and activates inositol-3-phosphate (increasing Ca^{2+}) and causing secretion and aggregation. The high-affinity site is thought to be reversible, and responsible for increasing intracellular Ca^{2+} and shape change. ADP has an important role in platelet aggregation following stimulation with TXA_2 via its release and resultant amplification response.

Glycoprotein IIb/IIIa receptors
The GPIIb/IIIa receptor is made up of two subunits α_{IIb} (CD41) and β_{III} (CD61), which are the products of separate genes that lie on the long arm of chromosome 17. It is the most abundant receptor present on the platelet surface at ~40 000–80 000 copies per cell. This represents the total number of fibrinogen-binding sites on the normal platelet. In addition, a pool of intracellular GPIIb/IIIa exists within the membranes of granules and can become expressed at the platelet surface in association with the secretory reaction. This can increase the number of functional receptors by 30–50%. In the

resting state, GPIIb/IIIa has a low affinity for circulating fibrinogen, but on activation it undergoes a conformational change and expresses a high-affinity binding site. Fibrinogen binds to GPIIb/IIIa receptors on multiple platelets, cross-linking them to form an aggregate. This process generates and releases further platelet agonists, and enhances the local activation and aggregation of platelets to form a stable platelet thrombus. This is often referred to as the final common pathway for platelet aggregation.

Thrombin receptors
Thrombin is central in the recruitment of platelets into the haemostatic plug at a site of vascular injury. Platelets possess protease-activated receptors which are activated by cleavage by thrombin and act via G-protein-linked mechanisms to cause platelet shape change, granule release and aggregation.

Antiplatelet drugs (Table 16.1)

Cyclooxygenase inhibitors: aspirin
Bayer released aspirin in 1899 for the treatment of fever and rheumatism, and just over 50 years later it was first suggested to reduce the risk of thrombotic arterial events. Aspirin is the most widely studied antiplatelet agent and it provides effective prophylaxis against vascular events. Aspirin is unique as it acts by irreversibly acetylating cyclooxygenase-1 and -2 (COX-1 and COX-2), thereby inhibiting TXA_2 and vasodilatory prostacyclin (prostaglandin I_2; PGI_2) formation. Endothelial cells are capable of regenerating COX, but platelets are anucleate and cannot regenerate this enzyme; therefore, the inhibitory action of aspirin on endothelial PGI_2 is transient, whereas its effect on platelets is permanent. Other NSAIDs have only a temporary inhibitory effect.

Platelets produce TXA_2 in response to various stimuli (including collagen, thrombin and ADP) and it has an important role in the amplification of platelet activation and vasoconstriction. However, reduced platelet activation by blockade of TXA_2 synthesis interferes with only one of the major secondary feedback loops for platelet activation and aggregation, and thrombosis can still occur in the presence of aspirin via other mechanisms. Aspirin is well absorbed, reaching a peak plasma level within 30 min of ingestion, and has a half-life of ~15–20 min. Studies demonstrated changes in platelet function within 1 h of ingestion, and bioavailability is good. Doses

Table 16.1 Antiplatelet agents

Mode of action	Antiplatelet drugs
Cyclooxygenase inhibitors	Aspirin, Ibuprofen, Indobufen, Sulphinpyrazone, Triflusal
Phosphodiesterase inhibitors	Dipyridamole, Cilostazol
Thromboxane synthase inhibitors	Picotamide
Thienopyridine derivatives	Ticlopidine, Clopidogrel, Prasugrel
Glycoprotein IIb/IIIa blockers	Abciximab, Eptifibatide, Tirofiban, Lamifiban, Xemilofiban and Orbofiba

of <300 mg daily appear to be as effective as higher doses, but with a lower risk of haemorrhagic or gastrointestinal side effects. In the UK, the standard dose used for thromboprophylaxis is 75–150 mg/day. Since aspirin is inexpensive and widely studied, it is the mainstay for antithrombotic prophylaxis in most guidelines. The Antithrombotic Trialists' Collaboration (a systematic review and meta-analysis) reported an ~25% risk reduction for cardiovascular events with the use of aspirin and that low-dose aspirin was as effective as higher doses.

Thromboxane synthase inhibitors: picotamide

This drug is a combined inhibitor of TXA_2 synthase and an antagonist of the TXA_2 receptors. It has been shown to reduce mortality in diabetics with PAD and lowers the risk of cardiovascular events in patients with acute myocardial infarction and previous ischaemic stroke. However, it is currently unavailable in many countries including the UK.

Thienopyridines: ADP receptor blockers

Clopidogrel and ticlopidine, thienopyridines, bind irreversibly to the platelet ADP ($P2Y_{12}$) receptor. Clopidogrel has now largely replaced ticlopidine in clinical practice as it has a more favourable side effect profile. Newer drugs such as prasugrel are currently being evaluated in clinical trials but are not licensed for use. There are some laboratory data and abundant anecdotal evidence that platelet function is more profoundly inhibited by clopidogrel than by aspirin. Clopidogrel is a 'pro-drug' activated in the liver, and the active metabolite is released for several days after the last oral dose (probably for 2–3 days). Thus, even transfused platelets may be ineffective in a patient who has taken oral clopidogrel within a few hours or days of a procedure. Elective surgery procedures should be delayed 7–10 days after stopping clopidogrel, by which time platelet function should be normal. The risk of stopping antiplatelet therapy should always be reviewed for each individual. The CAPRIE study compared clopidogrel with aspirin in patients with PAD, coronary disease or stroke. A relative risk reduction of 8.7% was obtained for clopidogrel (75 mg) versus aspirin (300 mg) overall, with subgroup *post hoc* analysis showing that the benefit was maximal in the PAD group. The UK NICE guidance is to use clopidogrel as a single agent in preference to aspirin only in those intolerant to aspirin. Intolerance is defined as a proven hypersensitivity or a history of severe indigestion caused by low-dose aspirin.

Phosphodiesterase inhibitors: dipyridamole and cilostazol

Dipyridamole is a pyrimidopyrimidine derivative that inhibits cyclic nucleotide phosphodiesterases and blocks the uptake of adenosine. This reduces cytosolic platelet Ca^{2+} concentration, and thereby inhibits platelet activation. Its effectiveness has not been proven as a sole antiplatelet agent in PAD. Its current clinical role is mainly in combination with aspirin in patients with recurrent cerebrovascular events. Cilostazol is licensed for the treatment of claudication in PAD. Its antiplatelet effects are relatively weak and it is not licensed for use in cardiovascular prophylaxis in the UK.

GPIIb/IIIa receptor blockers

Blocking the receptor (GPIIb/IIIa) responsible for fibrinogen binding is an effective and powerful method of preventing platelet aggregation.

Abciximab

The monoclonal antibody abciximab is directed against the active site of GPIIb/IIIa. This agent has undergone extensive clinical evaluation, and was the first agent in this class available for clinical use. It is licensed for use as an adjunct to aspirin and heparin in high-risk patients undergoing percutaneous coronary interventions (PCIs).

Eptifibatide and tirofiban

These also block the GPIIb/IIIa receptor and are used as adjuncts to aspirin and heparin to prevent myocardial infarction in patients with unstable angina or non-ST elevation myocardial infarction.

Despite their proven use in coronary disease, GPIIb/IIIa blockers have yet to establish a role in PAD particularly with their risks of adverse bleeding. Oral preparations are yet to prove effective.

Combination antiplatelet therapy

Combination antiplatelet therapy has evolved in the quest for more effective antiplatelet cover. However, guidelines vary widely between countries. The agents most commonly used are aspirin in combination with either clopidogrel or dipyridamole. NICE, based on analysis of cost-effectiveness, has recommended that patients with acute coronary syndromes—who do not undergo PCI—should be prescribed clopidogrel and aspirin for 12 months, after coronary stenting with a bare metal stent for 1 month and after drug-eluting stents for 12 months. For ST-elevation myocardial infarction the combination is used for 1 month.

In cerebrovascular disease, the European Stroke Prevention-2 trial of 6602 patients with prior stroke or TIA and the ESPRIT trial of 2739 patients found the combination of aspirin and dipyridamole to be more effective in reducing risk of further stroke or death compared with aspirin alone. Following ischaemic stroke or TIA, NICE recommend the combination of modified-release dipyridamole and aspirin for 2 years. In the MATCH trial of aspirin and clopidogrel versus clopidogrel alone in recent stroke or TIA, there was a non-significant benefit but an increase in life-threatening or major bleeding. However, clopidogrel as a solo agent is recommended for those intolerant of low-dose aspirin.

In PAD there are currently no strong data to prove the benefit of combination antiplatelet therapy. The CHARISMA study of the combination of aspirin and clopidogrel found no statistically significant benefit over aspirin treatment alone in a range of patients with established atherosclerotic disease including PAD.

Antiplatelet resistance (Box 16.1)

Despite antiplatelet therapy with aspirin, ~25% of patients will go on to have further vascular events. In addition, a wide range of platelet activity exists in patients taking aspirin when measured in

---

Box 16.1 **Causes of antiplatelet resistance**

- Drug non-compliance
- Variations in the pharmacokinetics and dynamics of aspirin metabolism (COX enzymatic activity, NSAID interactions)
- Platelet hyperactivity
- Primary (platelet receptor polymorphisms)
- Secondary (smoking, atherosclerosis, hyperlipidaemia)
- Methodological (variations in methods used to assess platelet function)

---

the laboratory by several techniques, including aggregation and flow cytometry. These observations led to the acceptance that certain people may be relatively resistant to the effects of aspirin ('aspirin resistance'), now extended to include other agents (anti-platelet resistance). The problem with the concept of aspirin resistance is that no clear definition exists. Definitions tend to fall either into clinical categories where vascular events occur despite aspirin, or into physiological categories where there is evidence of platelet hyperactivity on laboratory testing. Unfortunately, no reliable method currently exists that is suitable for assessing an individual's platelet aggregation response to antiplatelet therapy in a clinical context to allow 'tailoring' of doses or agents. Nevertheless, identification of aspirin non-responders has potentially important implications. This is an active area of research.

Conclusions

There is strong evidence that all patients with occlusive vascular disease (including PAD) should be on an antiplatelet agent, for prophylaxis against future events. Current guidelines in the UK from NICE recommend aspirin as first choice and clopidogrel as second line in patients who cannot take aspirin. Combination therapy is used for patients with acute coronary syndromes, following PCIs and after stroke or TIA. It is likely that in the future other high-risk subgroups, including those with multisite vascular disease, or aspirin resistance, may also be shown to benefit from combination treatment.

Further reading

Andrews RK, Berndt MC. Platelet physiology and thrombosis. *Thromb Res* 2004;**114**:447–453.

Antiplatelet Trialists' Collaboration. Collaborative meta-analysis of randomized trials of antiplatelet therapy for prevention of death, myocardial infarction, and stroke in high risk patients. *BMJ* 2002;**324**:71–86.

Bhatt DL, Fox KA, Hacke W *et al.* Clopidogrel and aspirin versus aspirin alone for the prevention of atherothrombotic events. *N Engl J Med* 2006;**354**:1706–1717.

CAPRIE Steering Committee. A randomized, blinded, trial of clopidogrel versus aspirin in patients at risk of ischaemic events (CAPRIE). *Lancet* 1996;**348**:1329–1339.

Hankey GJ. Antiplatelet therapy for the prevention of recurrent stroke and other serious vascular events: a review of the clinical trial data and guidelines. *Curr Med Res Opin* 2007;**23**:1453–1462.

Hankey GJ, Eikelboom JW. Aspirin resistance. *Lancet* 2006;**367**:606–617.

Neri Serneri GG, Coccheri S, Marubini E *et al.* Picotamide, a combined inhibitor of thromboxane A2 synthase and receptor, reduces 2-year mortality in diabetics with peripheral arterial disease: the DAVID study. *Eur Heart J* 2004;**25**:1845–1852.

NICE. Acute coronary syndromes—clopidogrel, 2004. http://www.nice.org.uk/.

NICE. Vascular disease—clopidogrel and dipyridamole, 2005. http://www.nice.org.uk/.

Norgren L, Hiatt WR, Dormandy JA *et al.* Inter-society consensus for the management of peripheral arterial disease (TASC II). *J Vasc Surg* 2007;**45**(Suppl S):S5–S67.

CHAPTER 17

Anticoagulation in Venous Thrombosis

John Pasi

OVERVIEW

- The role of anticoagulation in venous thromboembolism (VTE) is to prevent thrombus extension and recurrence.
- Initial treatment using low molecular weight heparin therapy is as efficacious as unfractionated heparins and has a number of clinical advantages.
- Warfarin has a very narrow therapeutic window and many important drug interactions.
- Secondary prevention of VTE and longer term anticoagulation with warfarin requires careful monitoring to ensure patient safety and that the international normalized ratio (INR) remains therapeutic.
- The duration and intensity of long-term anticoagulation is an area of controversy.

Anticoagulation therapy is the mainstay of treatment for venous thromboembolism (VTE), which encompasses deep-vein thrombosis (DVT) and pulmonary embolism (PE). Treatment regimens for DVT and PE are similar because the two conditions are manifestations of the same disease process. Anticoagulant therapy has two roles: initial treatment to prevent thrombus extension and long-term therapy to prevent recurrences of DVT and PE.

Although the initial data upon which anticoagulant therapy is based are now >40 years old, there continues to be much work in this area to look at the duration, intensity and safety of anticoagulation; anticoagulation has a relatively low therapeutic window, with both the benefits (reduced risk of thrombosis) and risks of anticoagulation (increased incidence of bleeding) being positively associated with both duration of treatment and degree of anticoagulation.

Heparin

Heparin is a sulphated glycosaminoglycan isolated from the intestinal mucosa or lung tissue. A specific five-sugar (pentasaccharide)

sequence in heparin binds tightly to antithrombin inducing a conformational change that results in increased inhibitory activity (~5000-fold) of antithrombin towards coagulation serine proteases such as thrombin (IIa), Xa and IXa.

Heparin is widely used as an anticoagulant both therapeutically and prophylactically. It has a rapid onset of action and a short half-life but can only be administered parenterally as it is rapidly destroyed by enzymes within the gut.

In an unfractionated form, heparin consists of chains of varying molecular weights (range 3000–30 000 Da, mean 15 000 Da). Heparin can be fractionated enzymatically or chemically cleaved to enrich for smaller, low molecular weight species (mean molecular weight 5000 Da). Whereas unfractionated heparin (UFH) has similar anti-Xa and anti-IIa activity, LMWHs have relatively greater anti-Xa activity. This is because there are fewer longer species that are required to cross-link the heparin–antithrombin complex to thrombin (see Figure 17.1).

Unfractionated heparin

Conventionally UFH is given therapeutically by continuous i.v. infusion or s.c. injection. The anticoagulant action is monitored by measuring the activated partial thromboplastin time (APTT) 4–6 h after starting treatment. The dose of heparin should be adjusted to maintain the APTT at 1.5–2.5 times the mid-point of the normal range.

Heparins have a great capacity to bind non-specifically to many plasma proteins, and the pharmacokinetics of UFH are dose dependent. These components vary significantly between individuals and with time. APTT is a global coagulation test and not specific for heparin—measuring plasma heparin levels is more accurate but it is impractical and expensive.

Failure to achieve adequate anticoagulation is very common with the use of UFH. APTT ratios <1.5 during the first 2 days increase the risk of recurrent VTE. APTT should be monitored every 6 h until the APTT is stable (i.e. at least first 24 h) and checked at least twice daily once stable.

Oral anticoagulants may be started at the same time (see below). Heparin should generally be continued for 5–7 days—this is the time needed to obtain an adequate antithrombotic effect with oral anticoagulants (e.g. warfarin). Once the INR is >2.5 for two

ABC of Arterial & Venous Disease, 2nd edn. Edited by R. Donnelly and N. London.
© 2009 Blackwell Publishing Ltd. 9781405178891.

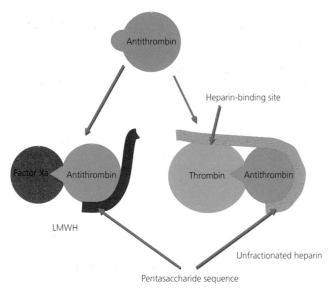

Figure 17.1 Heparins induce a conformational change in antithrombin, increasing inhibitory activity. However, only long heparin chains (at least 18 saccharide units) can complex antithrombin to thrombin

---

Box 17.1 **Mangement protocol for unfractionated heparin infusion**

- Measure baseline APTT, PT and platelet count
- Ensure no contraindications to the heparin
- Bolus dose of 5000 U (75 U/kg) heparin followed by an i.v infusion of 18 U/kg/h
- Check APTT after 4–6 h with adjustment of the dose if required and at least 6 hourly in first 24 h
- Repeat APTT at ~4 h after any dose adjustment
- Check twice daily thereafter
- Target APPT ratio 1.5–2.5 times mid-point of normal range
- Check platelet count daily

---

consecutive days heparin can be stopped. In complex cases, heparin may be continued for longer (Box 17.1).

Low molecular weight heparins

LMWHs are smaller, more uniform in size, have reduced non-specific protein binding and are principally excreted by the kidney.

LMWHs are therefore more predictable in dose–response relationships compared with UFH. LMWHs have a longer half-life than UFH.

LMWHs are used as first-line therapy for uncomplicated DVT and PE: many trials and meta-analyses have shown that LMWHs are at least as effective as UFH for treatment of submassive PE and DVT, have at least equivalent safety profiles and have greater cost-effectiveness over UFH.

LMWH dose is calculated on a patient weight basis and they only need to be administered once or twice daily s.c. (dependent upon the preparation). No anticoagulant monitoring for dose adjustment is required, enabling uncomplicated VTE to be managed in many cases on an outpatient basis, so saving 4–5 days' admission per patient.

In those rare cases where monitoring may be required, the heparin level measured via the anti-Xa activity is used. As LMWHs are eliminated via the kidneys, caution and/or dose reduction need to be taken with renal impairment.

As with UFH, oral anticoagulants may be started at the same time and LMWH discontinued when the INR is >2.5 for two consecutive days.

There are limited data on the use of LMWHs for massive DVT or PE. Although there is no evidence that LMWHs are likely to be less effective, some clinicians consider UFH the treatment of choice because of clinical experience and rapidity of onset (Table 17.1).

Heparin-induced thrombocytopenia

A rare complication is heparin-induced thrombocytopenia (HIT). A mild fall in platelet count is common, beginning on the second or third day of treatment, but rarely does it fall to $<100\times10^9$/l. This distinguishes it from the important form of HIT where the platelet count may fall to much lower levels ($20–50\times10^9$/l) that is paradoxically associated with platelet thrombi and arterial and venous thrombosis. This rare complication is due to a platelet-activating antibody directed against platelet factor 4 (PF4) complexed to heparin. Typically HIT presents ≥5 days after exposure to heparin. Upon diagnosis, heparin must be stopped, but there remains a high risk of thrombosis which requires therapeutic anticoagulation. Warfarin should be delayed as it can lead to an increased risk of microvascular thrombosis. Alternatives to heparin include heparinods (danapaorid), recombinant hirudin or argatroban. HIT antibodies may persist for up to 6 weeks after the cessation of heparin.

Table 17.1 Comparision of unfractionated and low molecular weight heparins

Unfractionated heparin	Low molecular weight heparin
Increased half-life with increased concentration of drug (range 30 min to 4 h)	Stable half-life, ~4 h, and more predictable dose response
Non-specific protein binding	Reduced non-specific binding
<50% bioavailability subcutaneously (at low dosage)	>90% bioavailability subcutaneously
Monitoring required with APTT	No monitoring required (anti-Xa if occasionally needed)
Risk of HIT	Lower risk of HIT
Hepatic and renal elimination	Renal elimination

HIT = heparin-induced thrombocytopenia.

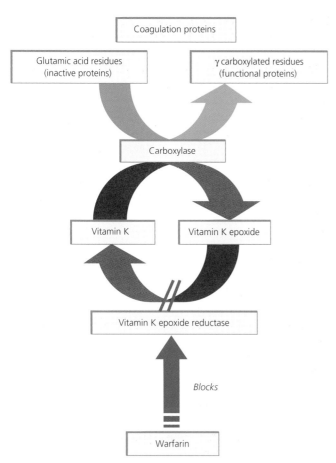

Figure 17.2 Warfarin inhibits vitamin K epoxide reductase so reducing functional coagulation protein synthesis

Oral anticoagulants

The most commonly used oral anticoagulant drug is warfarin—a coumarin. Warfarin inhibits metabolic pathways that are necessary for the gamma carboxylation of the vitamin K-dependent coagulant proteins (factors II, VII, IX, X, protein C and S). With such impaired post-translational modification these coagulation proteins are dysfunctional and hence warfarin produces an anticoagulant/antithrombotic effect. The antithrombotic effects of warfarin are mainly due to reduction in factor X and II levels (Figure 17.2).

Warfarin is well absorbed from the gastrointestinal tract and has high bioavailability. It is metabolized by hepatic cytochrome P450 complex and highly protein bound (99%+) in plasma. As a consequence it has many significant drug interactions. Other patient variables such as diet, compliance, concurrent illness, liver function and certain genetic variants may also significantly affect response to warfarin. Warfarin is a drug with a narrow therapeutic window and requires regular monitoring using the International Normalised Ratio (INR)—an internationally agreed index for control of anticoagulant therapy based upon the prothrombin time. Patients on warfarin must be systematically followed with regular INR testing and good patient communication of results and dosing decisions (Box 17.2).

Box 17.2 **Drugs and other factors that interfere with warfarin anticoagulation**

Inherited sensitivity (CYP2C9)/resistance (VKORC1) genes
Enhanced anticoagulation: acute illness, increasing age, impaired liver function, renal failure, excess alcohol, diet poor in vitamin K
Drugs
Enhanced anticoagulation:
- Reduced protein binding: aspirin, chlorpromazine, sulphonamides
- Inhibition of warfarin metabolism: cimetidine, allopurinol, tricyclic antidepressants, metronidazole, erythromycin, sodium valproate
- Reduced vitamin absorption: antibiotics, laxatives
- Decreased clotting factor synthesis: cephalosporins, phenytoin

Reduced anticoagulation:
- Increased metabolism of warfarin: barbiturates, rifampacin, carbamazepine
- Increased clotting factor synthesis: oral contraceptives

Warfarin is frequently started in conjunction with heparin (see above). Therapeutic anticoagulation is only achieved when the levels of factor II and X drop, which is generally after ~5 days of warfarin. Heparin can be stopped when the INR is consistently ≥2.5.

A target INR 2.0–3.0 is also generally satisfactory for treatment of DVT, PE and recurrent venous thrombosis if the recurrence occurred off anticoagulants. Higher target INR (3.0–4.5) is indicated for recurrent VTE occurring on anticoagulants and those with antiphospholipid syndrome.

The duration of therapy is indication dependent but usually for a first event of significance is ~3–6 months. Longer term treatment depends upon the clinical circumstances and risk of recurrence (Box 17.3).

Box 17.3 **Duration of anticoagulation**

Three to six months
- Calf vein thrombosis with no persistent risk factors
- DVT and PE in association with reversible (transient) risk factors

Six months to 1 year
- First event of PE or DVT (idiopathic)

Indefinite
- Antiphospholipid syndrome, PE or DVT in association with two or more thrombophilic risk factors, recurrent events (with or without thrombophilia), cancer (or until resolved)

Thrombophilia
- Evidence of an inherited thrombophilia lowers threshold for indefinite or longer term anticoagulation

Table 17.2 Reversal of oral anticoagulation

INR and symptoms	Action
3.0–6.0 (target INR 2.5)	Reduce warfarin dose or stop
4.0–6.0 (target INR 3.5)	Restart warfarin when INR < 5.0
6.0–8.0	
No bleeding or minor bleeding	Stop warfarin
	Restart warfarin when INR < 5.0
>8.0	Stop warfarin
No bleeding or minor bleeding	Restart warfarin when INR < 5.0
	If other risk factors for bleeding give 0.5–2.5 mg vitamin K
Major bleeding	Stop warfarin
	Give prothrombin complex concentrate 50 U/kg or FFP 15 ml/kg
	Give 5 mg vitamin K

FFP = fresh frozen plasma.
Adapted from British Committee for Standards in Haematology (1998).

When treatment is stopped, recurrent VTE occurs at a rate initially of ~5% per year, with an overall recurrence rate at 10 years of ~30%. There is a rationale for extended duration of therapy if the risk of major bleeding could be reduced from the current level of ~2% per annum. Recent studies have looked at prolonged anticoagulation, using a either a standard or a reduced INR target. — lowering the INR results in more recurrences with no advantage in terms of the risk of bleeding, compared with standard INR, but less recurrence compared with placebo. This, however, remains an area of some controversy.

Haemorrhage is the major side effect of warfarin. Significant bleeding, and indeed fatal bleeding events, may occur at therapeutic INRs, but the risks of bleeding increases dramatically with increasing INR (especially >5.0) and with increasing patient age. Dependent upon the severity of bleeding, options for treatment include simply stopping warfarin, vitamin K, fresh frozen plasma (FFP) or preferably prothrombin complex concentrates (Table 17.2).

Thrombolytic therapy

Theoretically, the use of thrombolytic agents (such as tissue plasminogen activator (tPA) and streptokinase) to lyse thrombi and clear venous obstruction would seem a rational approach for patients with VTE. However, the clinical importance of rapid clearance is uncertain. In addition thrombolytic agents increase the risk of bleeding. Use of thrombolytics is not recommended for uncomplicated VTE and is generally reserved for those with massive ileofemoral DVT at risk of limb gangrene or those with massive PE and haemodynamic instability (Box 17.4).

Inferior vena caval filters

The only purpose of an IVC filter is to prevent PE. The primary reason for use is a contraindication to or complication of antico-

Box 17.4 Treatment regimes for thrombolyis for massive PE

Assess suitability of patient for thrombolytic therapy
Select
- Streptokinase 250 000 IU loading dose followed by 100 000 IU/h for 2 h
or
- Urokinase 4400 IU/kg body weight loading dose followed by 2200 IU/kg for 12 h
or
- Recombinant tPA 100 mg infusion over 2 h (*preferred*)
Check APTT and fibrinogen 2–4 h after starting infusion—a reduction in fibrinogen and prolongation of APTT indicates active fibrinolysis
Commence heparin infusion when APTT ratio <2 and maintain at APTT ratio 1.5–2.5

agulation in those at high risk for recurrent PE. Anticoagulation should be resumed as soon as possible after filter insertion—filters alone are not an effective treatment of VTE.

IVC filters are not indicated in patients with VTE who would otherwise be on conventional anticoagulant therapy, albeit they may have a role in selected patients with PE despite high-intensity therapeutic anticoagulation or those with recent VTE (within 1 month) who require anticoagulation interruption (e.g. surgery).

Filters can be safely inserted via either the internal jugular or femoral veins under fluoroscopic guidance. They may be either permanent or temporary (retrievable)—retrievable filters should be used for patients with a short-term contraindication to anticoagulant therapy. IVC filters are associated with significant incidence of recurrent DVT and IVC thrombosis which appear not to be influenced by anticoagulant therapy (Fig. 17.3).

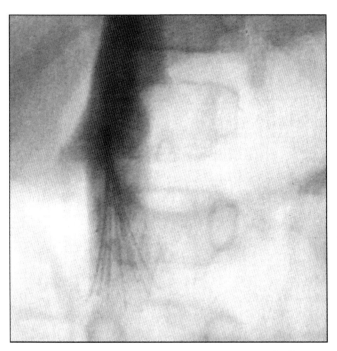

Figure 17.3 Vena cavagram showing umbrella delivery device for filter inserted into the inferior vena cava through the jugular vein (as per previous ABC , BMJ 325: p950 – photo of vena caval filter)

Treatment during pregnancy

VTE in pregnancy can be safely treated with heparins—heparins (UFH and LMWH) do not cross the placenta and are the anticoagulant of choice for prevention and treatment of pregnancy-associated VTE. Warfarin, however, is teratogenic and should not be given in pregnancy.

Cancer-associated VTE

VTE in cancer is associated with a poorer outcome, more recurrent VTE and more bleeding complications due to anticoagulant therapy. Although warfarin is the standard of care for secondary prevention of VTE, in the cancer setting it is associated with a higher rate of recurrent VTE than use of LMWH. Increasingly LMWH is recommended as the treatment of choice for cancer-associated VTE until the cancer is resolved.

Novel orally active anticoagulants

Considerable pharmaceutical research is currently underway investigating novel anticoagulant drugs that could replace warfarin. These drugs fall into two main classes—direct thrombin inhibitors (e.g. dabigitran) and anti-Xa inhibitors (e.g. rivaroxaban). Such drugs have been developed to provide a significantly wider therapeutic window than warfarin, so offering fixed dosing, fewer significant drug or dietary interactions and no need for monitoring of anticoagulant effect. Data on their safety and efficacy in VTE are awaited, but, if encouraging, these would be very promising compounds that could significantly reduce the patient burden of being on warfarin.

Further reading

Baglin T, Barrowcliffe TW, Cohen A, Greaves M, the British Committee for Standards in Haematology. Guidelines on the use and monitoring of heparin. *Br J Haematol* 2006;**133**:19–34.

Baglin TP, Brush J, Streiff M, the British Committee for Standards in Haematology. Guidelines on use of vena cava filters. *Br J Haematol* 2006;**134**:590–595.

Baglin TP, Keeling DM, Watson HG, the British Committee for Standards in Haematology. Guidelines on oral anticoagulation (warfarin): third edition—2005 update. *Br J Haematol* 2006;**132**:277–285.

British Committee for Standards in Haematology. Guidelines on oral anticoagulation: third edition *Br J Haematol* 1998;**101**:374–387.

Kearon C, Kahu SR, Agnelli G, *et al.* Antithrombotic Therapy for Venous Thromboembolic Disease: American College of Chest Physicians Evidence-based Clinical Practice Guidelines (8th Edition) *Chest* 2008;**133**:454S–545S

Index